Messy Bed, Messy Head

Messy Bed, Messy Head

Where Clutter Comes From
& How To Clean It Up

Cindy L. Cooley

Published 2019

KDP ISBN: 9781797945743
ASIN: B07L52M2RZ

Cover Photo: Licensed through DepositPhotos.com ©photographee.eu
Cover Designer: Stephanie Hannus
Managing Editor: Bethany Davis
Proofreader/Editor: Sarah Cisco
Author's photo courtesy of Kim Forman, Kimfluence Photography

Dedicated to Scott, my love, for...EVERYTHING!

Table of Contents

Acknowledgements

"Next to excellence is the appreciation of it."
~William Makepeace Thackeray

Just as it's true that no composer coughs up a masterpiece in one sitting, no scientist discovers the origins of a problem and saves humanity with a single theory, it is also true that no writer births a book without a cadre of midwives and doulas to assist them in the process. Please indulge me as I take a moment to acknowledge and honor the amazing people who enrich my life, and made this book possible.

On a professional level, first and foremost, I'd like to thank Dr. Angela Lauria, the amazing powerhouse behind The Author Incubator Program, who created a process that allowed me to go from concept to finished rough draft in nine of the single most transformative weeks of my life. Not only did I go from concept to finished rough draft in a mercifully brief period of time under Angela's tutelage, but she introduced me to my inner author, and gave the books lined-up inside me a path into the world. Thank you, Angela!

Angela doesn't work her considerable magic in a vacuum. She has a fantastic team supporting her without whom *Messy Bed, Messy Head* would've been much less coherent and cohesive...

Cheyenne Giesecke, without her gentle yet super-efficient touch organizing, coordinating, and guiding all the moving parts of the program, I fear it would...shudder...let's not even go there! Thank you, Cheyenne!

Ora North, developmental editor extraordinaire, who gave my nebulous thoughts shape and form. Such a gentle soul, yet able to make you go back and redo something again and again until you get it right, while smiling and encouraging you all the while. Thank you, Ora!

Bethany Davis, magnificent managing editor, who has the gift of making a budding author feel like her words matter, and that she was created to make a difference in this world. She showed me how less really can be more effective. Thank you, Bethany!

There are more members of her team who deserve special mention, for sure, but suffice to say that the whole Author Incubator team have a philosophy of building their writer's up rather than tearing them down. They hold space for their author's growth, and I adore each and every one of them.

Once the edits of my rough draft were complete, Bethany suggested I consider the website Reedsy to find a proofreader and cover designer. Best. Advice. Ever.

I hired Sarah Cisco as a proofreader from Reedsy. She is knowledgeable and professional, and went so far above and beyond the call of duty that she deserves extra mention here. If there are any mistakes in this book it is because I fluffed, and stuffed, and tweaked things after her final look-see. Thank you, Sarah!

Also through Reedsy, I found Stephanie Hannus, who took my vague vision and created cover art that invites the reader to curl up in their favorite chair and spend an afternoon opening their heart and mind. Again, like my proofreader, she went above and beyond with creativity, integrity, and an incredible work ethic. Thank you, Stephanie!

The lesson for all self-published authors: if you want to be taken seriously as a professional writer, act like one. Invest in your work, your vision, your book, and yourself by hiring a team of professionals to support you.

On a more personal level, I am who I am because of the incredible family and friends I'm surround by.

My children, Joshua, Tyler, and Paige, have had to bear the brunt of being raised by a mother desperately trying to get her shit together yet coming up short time and time again. That they are wonderful, beautiful human beings is more a testament to their extraordinary Divine selves than it is to me as their mother.

My five grandchildren: Beau (Sugar Booger), Peyton (Peyton Pie), Hunter (Honey Bunny), Bella (Bella Boo-Boo), and Emily Grace (Love Bug). I get teary-eyed just thinking of the blessing they are to me. Children are a responsibility that force you to become the best version of yourself. Grandchildren are like frosting, or gravy, that make life yummy and sweet, and so very worthwhile.

To Maggie and Brandie, the mothers of my grandchildren. I cannot thank you enough for the precious gifts you've given me.

To my mother and my father, I am who I am because you are my parents. If I blame you for the things you did that fucked me and my siblings up, I must also thank you for the role you played in creating a woman who is kind, compassionate, and can handle hard things. Without you both, I wouldn't be as awesome as I am. I don't need anything in my life to be any different than it is, and I am grateful that you are my parents. I love you, and thank you both.

To my sister Celena and my brother Clint, there is nobody else I could've survived our childhood with, but you two. At a very young age, we were ripped apart, scattered to the wind, and thrown to the wolves, and yet...still we stand strong, and can handle anything life throws our way. Few can understand us like we understand each other. I love you both.

I am blessed with great friends, but Kim Forman is my BFF, and heterosexual life partner. Imagine having a friend who ALWAYS has your back. One you can laugh with, cry with, vent with, who is your biggest cheerleader, and thinks every harebrained idea you have is a fantastic idea you are sure to succeed at with undiminished enthusiasm – no matter how many you've had – and who never rubs your nose in it when they don't work out, or you get distracted by the next super duper brilliant harebrained idea. Our friendship is such a blessing to me. I love you to the moon and back, Swirlygrrl!

I saved the best for last. Scott Cooley...my love, my life, my husband, the man I love so much I married him twice. We have been through everything together: life, death, birth, loss, desolation, desperation, hope, growth, love, laughter, peace, prosperity, marriage, and even divorce. Amidst my periods of chaos and clutter, you see my beauty and love me no matter what. I love you, Scotty, and am so happy that the universe made us for each other!

Chapter 1 – You're Not Broken

"Stop trying to 'fix' yourself;
you're NOT broken!
You are perfectly imperfect and
powerful beyond measure."
~Stephen Maraboli

There are women who seem to breeze through life, career, motherhood, and marriage with grace and ease. Their homes are always spotless, their children's play clothes have been ironed, their husbands worship the ground they walk on, and their careers are sexy and rewarding. I am not one of them, and I'm guessing, if this book appeals to you, neither are you.

My children had clean clothes to wear to school, but, more times than not, they pulled them out of a basket because they hadn't been folded, or put away yet...and probably never would. And yes, they've certainly had to wash a glass to get a drink because all the glasses were dirty.

When I became a mother, I swore that would never happen with my children. I swore I'd be a better mother than the one I had, but life gets in the way, and overwhelm soon sets in, doesn't it?

Soon after clutter and chaos take over your life, isolation sets in. You can't stand for people who know and love you to see your house like this, so you put space between you and them, and avoid them. The pain of losing friends is bearable because the pain of facing your own perceived failure is worse.

Better not to think too much about it. Easier not to feel too much.

Over the years, there's a part of you that shuts down when you don't meet your own ideals. It makes the overwhelm easier to deal with if you don't have to wallow in it constantly. It's like going to sleep, and, if you're not careful, decades can race past you in this zombie-like state.

But, one day, something happens to snap you out of the anesthetized stupor…

Your child wants to have friends over to play, and you hear the friend tell your child they can't come inside to play because their mom said your house is too dirty. A part of you bristles, "How would she know, she's never set foot in here." But then you look around at the dirty dishes covering almost every available inch of counter space, the laundry that seems to have grown legs and moves and multiplies at will, and the overflowing trash can that everybody in your household tries to pile as high as possible without toppling it, like a weird version of Jenga.

Or, perhaps you read something, or see something on TV, that jolts you to your core and forces you to look at the life you've created for yourself, your husband, and your children. There is a deeper part of you trying to get your attention, and, in that moment of awakening, you feel it cry out.

You'd like to go back to sleep, but you can't, and you are struck with the certainty that something must change, and the only variable under your control…the only thing that can possibly change…is you.

The real question is, how do you change? How do you think different thoughts? How do you feel different feelings? How do you believe different beliefs? How do you take different actions? How do you transform a life of habituated disempowering behavior that keeps you and your family drowning in chaos and clutter, into a life of happiness and fulfillment? *Messy Bed, Messy Head* is all about giving you the tools you need to change your beliefs, change your thinking, and change your emotions that keep you from taking action to create the home you and your family can be proud of.

There are so many young mothers who've never had someone show them how to make a bed, create a schedule, deliberately create empowering rituals/habits that govern their days, or create order in their lives. Increasingly, Americans look to YouTube University to answer questions our parents never taught us. We don't know what to do, so we're also raising children with no responsibilities, and no work ethic. Not because we don't want to, but most of us just don't know how. It's no wonder everyone feels like the world is spinning out of control, and they have no clue where the steering wheel is, much less how to grab ahold to take control!

You are not broken. You are not alone. There are many, many women who struggle with the overwhelm and get buried beneath the avalanche, and never-ending onslaught of clutter, just like you. You've simply created, or been handed, a series of disempowering habits, and habits can be changed. Throughout this book, I'll show you how.

Motivation Fallacy

I'm not sure where it came from, but I'd like to bitch-slap the person who hypnotized our society into believing you had to be *motivated* to start something. Motivation is the single most useless spark for starting a creative fire. Utterly useless.

In his magnificent book, *The Motivation Myth: How High Achievers Really Set Themselves Up To Win*, author Jeff Haden says that motivation is actually the result of achievement, not the impetus to start a project in the first place. Small wins build the momentum that result in motivation, not the other way around.

I share this with you because if you wait for motivation to strike before you get a handle on the clutter and chaos inside your home, you'll grow old and die first. There are exercises in this book that can help you gain a treasure trove of small wins and get your motivation engine fired up!

Benefits Of Decluttering

There are many benefits to cleaning, decluttering, and organizing for you and your family:

- Safety
- Health
- Clarity
- Order
- It creates a framework, a structure to manage your environment
- It sets the energetic tone for your home and releases energetic drains
- It releases pent-up creative energy.

It's all possible. You can have order and clarity. You can have structure and ritual. You can manage your time, master your environment, and own your creativity.

With time and attention, and a series of 10-minute tasks that create a sense of small wins, you can create an environment that puts people at ease the moment they walk into your home. Your children can have friends come over to play and forget they were ever embarrassed to ask someone to come inside. By understanding, and tweaking, some of your most basic habits, your home can be an inviting oasis of calm.

I know what you're going through; I've been there and found a way through the chaos and clutter to order and clarity. The guilt, the shame, the embarrassment, the frustration, the resentment, and the resignation into mediocrity that have become your constant companions don't have to overwhelm you anymore.

Let me show you how...

Chapter 2 – Growing Up Messy

"It's your reaction to adversity, not adversity itself,
that determines how your life story will develop."
~Dieter F. Uchtforf

You can make anything normal. Chaos? Clutter? Yeah, anything.

When you're born into a mess and raised in a mess, you don't know there's another way until you get into grade school, and realize that other kids don't live the same way you do.

As human beings, we are all shades of light and dark, beauty and ugliness, and as such, we are capable of generating the most magnificent dreams, or the most horrific nightmares. Every single one of us.

My mother is no exception. As a child, I grew up knowing that she loved me completely, and never doubted it. She thought I was wonderful, independent, and instilled me with a sense that I was special, blessed, and capable of absolutely anything. That was her light. Her darkness? My mother wasn't a hoarder, per se, she just never took out the trash, did the laundry, or cleaned. Ever.

To be a true hoarder, in the pathological sense, is to imbue junk with intrinsic value and stockpile it away for the future as if it were a treasure of sorts. I don't know if there is a word, or diagnosis, for someone who is simply too lazy to get up and put trash in a garbage can, make a bed, give a child a bath, or wash a dish, but that would certainly apply to my mother.

She probably never should've had children. She told me on many occasions how much she hated anything that smacked of taking care of *others*, which included her family. She dreamt of being in the Navy, or being a truck driver – typically masculine things – anything but a wife and mother.

Until I was eight years old, I grew up in a traditional, dysfunctional nuclear-family dynamic: mother, father, three children (in birth order, I am the baby), an odd assortment of pets that never stayed for very long, and clothes, dishes, and trash strewn everywhere. And by everywhere, I mean behind the couch, randomly scattered on the floor, under the bed, in the garage, or next to the garbage can. You couldn't even see the bathroom floor for all the damp, mildew-ridden, moldy, urine-stained clothes.

What was dirty, or clean? Impossible to tell.

Every available countertop was filled with dirty dishes, so, if you were thirsty, you had to wash a glass before you could drink. My sister, who is six years older than I, remembers brushing cockroaches out of her hair before going to school, and was always terrified a bug would fall out of her hair in the middle of class.

While I'm sure there were times my mother cleaned up, I honestly cannot remember a single one.

If you thought our house was bad, the garage was even worse. Bags of trash thrown into the garage instead of taken to the road sat atop months' (if not years') worth of rotting garbage. It literally smelled like the town dump, and so did we.

My mother and father fought constantly, bitterly over the filthy state of our house. In the end, after 15 years of marriage, they hated each other so much that, more than 45 years later, they can't even be in the same state with each other at the same time. Joint presences at graduations, marriages, or births are an absolute no-no, and it is far more likely that neither will show up. Neither of my parents attended my wedding, my college graduation, or even the births of my children.

One of my earliest memories was going to my Grandma Kiddoo's house and being amazed at how tidy everything was. You didn't have to move trash out of the way to sit down. You didn't have to nudge dirty dishes aside to get to the sink, or wash a glass so you could get a drink of milk, and there was no possibility that the milk was...chunky.

My grandma and grandpa lived in Kansas. We lived in Missouri. I remember crying when we left to go back home because I didn't want to leave.

Our house had a huge mulberry tree in the backyard. I loved to climb up to the highest branch I could lay on, pick and eat mulberries, and stare up at the sky daydreaming. It smelled sweet, woody, and clean. To this day, I love the smell of mulberries. I can drive down a road in a town I've never been in, and know there are mulberry trees in bloom somewhere around me just from their scent wafting on the breeze.

~~~~~

I was three or four years old when our house burnt to the ground. All the years' worth of rotting trash and piles of old newspapers in the garage got too close to the gas water heater and caught on fire.

There is something both sad and disturbing about walking through a pile of rubble that used to be your home. Debris hangs in the air, and it's impossible to distinguish the clouds of ash kicked up from your steps as you trudge through the rubble from the smoke. Seeing the piles of garbage and clothes rendered to ash. The acrid stench of burnt wood and cotton and Naugahyde – and melted aluminum pots and pans and rotten trash – assault your nostrils. I caught sight of a singed and blackened ear, arm, and leg, which were all that was left of my favorite stuffed bunny.

I remember being terrified, but also happy and excited when I saw the rubble because my mom and dad were discussing how we'd have to find someplace else to live.

In his seminal coaching program *Personal Power II*, Tony Robbins repeatedly says, "The problem with thinking something, someone, or someplace else will be better than what you've got right now is that you take *you* with you." I was too young to realize it wasn't just the house that was dirty, it was us too.

There is a weird time/memory dysmorphia thing that happens when you're very young and grow up a child of filth and chaos. Time from my youth doesn't move in a linear fashion for me. Until I turned eight, time was broken up into highly emotional chunks of events.

For instance, to the best of my recollection, we moved from Missouri to Arizona around the time our house burnt down, but I can't remember if it was because our house burned down and we had nowhere else to go, or because my parents were running from creditors and the occasional enraged bookie, or some combination thereof.

~ ~ ~ ~ ~

When I think back on my grandmothers, both of them, I know how fortunate I am to have grown up with them looking out for me. They are proof that the Universe has my back.

My father's mother, Grandma Kiddoo, was intelligent, wise, meticulous, and embodied grace. She was the only person who really "got" me. At just under six foot, she was a tall woman with black hair, and black eyes that never flickered or flinched and flashed with keen insight and intelligence. This was always interesting to me because I don't believe she made it in school much past the 6th grade, but she was the most intelligent person I knew.

Grandma Kiddoo had her first child when she was barely a child herself. Her first husband was horribly abusive, so she, a young teenage mother, left him during the Great Depression and raised her son by taking in laundry and cleaning other people's houses. There was no time for school, much less a higher education, yet she grasped complicated subjects with ease.

She was meticulous in nature, would never consider leaving the house unless she had her hair and makeup done, the bed made, the house cleaned, and she always dressed like she was going to church. Grandma Kiddoo had morning and evening rituals around cleaning her home and getting herself ready.

She was the mother of four boys, my father being second in the birth order, so you couldn't get away with anything in her presence. It's like she could see into your soul and know your deepest thoughts. I was smart, and she made me promise to go to college, which, while I didn't start until I was in my 30s – over a decade after her death – and didn't graduate until I was in my 40s, I did earn my BA in Creative Writing because I promised her I would.

She was a smart, capable, and wise woman who saw life as a classroom and the obstacles she faced as gifts to help her evolve into the best version of herself possible. Domestic violence, lack of a formal education, being an unapologetic divorcee in an era when divorce was unheard of, and she faced it all with dignity and grace. Grandma Kiddoo lived a life so hard she even had to live in a chicken coop for a while – which she kept meticulously clean – after she was widowed by her second husband (my grandfather), leaving her alone to raise four little boys during the Great Depression and World War II.

The mantras that guided her life were, "Experience is the BEST teacher" and "Soap is cheap, there is no excuse for filthiness."

As I write this, I cannot imagine how difficult it was for my father to go from having this meticulous woman as his mother to my messy, incredibly needy mother as his wife. Talk about extreme opposites!

Grandma Kiddoo taught me that the darkness comes bearing gifts, and there is nothing life throws at you that you cannot handle and be better because of – nothing – and that putting my house and self in order put my mind in order too.

~~~~~

My mother was from Arizona, my father was from Kansas, and I knew I had other grandparents living in Arizona but had no memory of them until we moved there when I was five-ish. My mother and her mother had a falling out years earlier, and momma had not a kind word to say about her. Her lips would pucker into a sneer of displeasure whenever she spoke about her mother, which said far more than her lack of kind words ever did.

I remember meeting my Grandma Wright for the first time after we moved to Arizona. She lived in a town 150 miles from us, and I was amazed that she drove all that way just to see us.

Because of the disapproving way my mother spoke about her own mother, I fully expected a monster to get out of the car when she pulled up to the curb. But monsters don't drive three hours just to see their grandchildren, do they? I pictured her with wiry grey hair poking up in every direction, hairy warts on her nose and chin, and no teeth...or maybe just one or two rotten teeth, at most.

Instead, out came a petite woman with a glorious crown of silver hair that glowed in the sunlight like a halo, and sparkling blue eyes that danced with merriment and delight. She scooped me up in a hug so full of love and longing and joy that I fell instantly in love with her.

Grandma Wright, my mother's mother, was kind, playful, genteel, tidy, and poised. She was a true lady, in every sense of the word, and, far from the monster I feared, was the kindest, gentlest human being I have ever known.

Like Grandma Kiddoo, Grandma Wright had cleaning and organizing rituals that governed her mornings and evenings, and, as she often said, "Put her mind in order."

Honestly, when I was a little child, I didn't spend a lot of time pining for a clean house because I spent as much time as I could outdoors. I was a wild child, a free spirit. The moment I was allowed to cross the street by myself, I spent as much time as I could outside. I fell in love with nature, and nature fell in love with me. Plants and animals pulse with life-force energy that I can feel. To this day, being cooped up in a house feels punishing to me.

It wasn't until I entered school that I knew I was different from other children. I remember the humiliation I felt the first time my friend told me she couldn't come to my house anymore because her mother said it was too dirty. I also remember the second, third...fifth...and tenth times too, and the moment I stopped asking childhood playmates to come over altogether. I remember the pinched look of disgust on my first-grade teacher's face when she sniffed my hair and suggested I needed a bath. To this day, I am hyper-conscious of unpleasant odors and all about smelling clean. (Until I wrote this, I had no idea why my body's scents are so important to me, but I'll talk more about this in Chapter 12, "Explore Your Mindset," and how you can use these deeply ingrained patterns within yourself to change literally anything you want to change about yourself.)

My life changed drastically when I turned eight because my parents divorced. Within a week of their divorce being final, my mother remarried (a story for another book), and soon after that, my mother, stepfather, brother, and I moved to my mother's hometown in Northwestern Arizona. (My sister stayed with our father 150 miles away.)

While I missed my father and sister horribly, our house wasn't disgustingly filthy anymore. Oh, it wasn't exactly clean – dishes and laundry would still pile up from time to time – but trash didn't accumulate in mounds, nor did you have to wade through it to get to the bathroom.

It's not because my mother had a change of heart and suddenly turned into Betty Crocker. Not at all. It was because my stepfather refused to live in a pigsty, so he took out the trash, and mostly cooked.

From that time forward, my mother's house went through phases of clutter and disarray that ranged from light to heavy, but the abject filth I was born into, and spent the first eight years of my life living in, was a thing of the past.

It felt like the Universe spared me from one form of chaos only to be plunged into another, which was, in many ways, worse. Far worse.

~~~~~

My stepfather may have taken the trash out on the regular, but it was usually because it was full of beer cans. He was a drunk, and a mean one at that (yet another story for another book.)

We moved into a house just on the other side of the hill from my Grandma Wright. I thought it odd that we lived only four blocks away from her but she never came to our house. Never. Not once. But, she didn't have to because I was ALWAYS at her house anyway.

In the morning, I would jump out of bed and run over the hill so she could fix me breakfast and French braid my hair before school. Her house was clean and tidy – no dust gathered on her knick-knacks or baseboards – and so well organized. I liked to pretend I lived with her and followed her around from room to room as she literally, and metaphorically, put her house in order.

Like Grandma Kiddoo, Grandma Wright never left her house without her hair and makeup done, and she always looked like she was going to church too.

One morning, I asked her why she went to all the bother of making her bed when she was just going to crawl back in it every night, and she told me, "Messy bed, messy head!"

When I asked her to elaborate, she pointed to her head and said, "Everything you see around you is a reflection of what's going on in here. If I left things undone they'd pile up, and I wouldn't be able to think straight."

Grandma Wright was gentle on the outside, but had a spine of steel like most of the women who came of age during the Great Depression. I was so proud to be her "official helper." My education in homemaking came from her. She taught me how to make a bed, cook, wash, rinse, and dry dishes, and how to do laundry – everything from sorting (why you shouldn't wash white clothes with red, or towels with sheets) to washing (how to hang them on the line to dry, iron, fold, and put away.)

From the tender age of 10, I did my own laundry, bathed on a daily basis, and made my bed. My brother and I shared a room, and my corner was an oasis of calm amidst the clutter and chaos that would collect in the rest of the house. I loved smelling clean, and it delighted me to see the smooth expanse of covers, orderly piles of socks and panties in their drawers, and clothes hung in order from skirts, capris, pants, sleeveless shirts, short sleeves, ¾ length sleeves, long sleeves, and dresses. And to this day, I love to iron. I even iron my sheets. Very Zen!

Truth be told, throughout the years, I may not have made my bed when I first got up, but at some point during the day – even if it was right before I crawled beneath the covers to sleep (drove my husband insane!) – my bed got made.

Carrying On The Family Tradition

I would love to say that my sojourn through chaos ended there, but that would be a lie.

Every one of you has a battle you must fight in order to express the best version of yourselves. Every. Single. One. Mine, without a doubt, are chaos, clutter, disorder, and obesity, which I strongly suspect are somehow linked.

Growing up a child of chaos has consequences for children that are inflicted upon them by their parents. Those who grow up with clutter and disarray as constant companions will crave stability and structure in order to feel safe and protected, yet their raising also makes stability and self-discipline two things they will have to fight to learn and create for themselves.

In one form or another, clutter and chaos have been my companions during this lifetime. So much so that, if things are going too smoothly, I've been known to blow my life up just to have a mess to clean up (perhaps another book.)

And I do love to clean up messiness. Thanks to my grandmothers, I entered young womanhood knowing exactly how to do that.

However...

~ ~ ~ ~ ~

Two events in my late teens knocked me sideways, and, in many ways, I've only recently recovered from them. I don't want to go into super detail on those events because it's *not* the events themselves, but my inability to deal with them effectively that set a chain of events into motion that buried me in layers of fat, and my own children in clutter and chaos, for years.

The day after my 17th birthday, my stepfather attacked me. I cannot say he tried to rape me, but I cannot say he didn't either. When all was said and done, my mother, who was my whole world, kicked me out of the house and threw me to the wolves, leaving me as prey to unscrupulous people. The following year, at 18, I was attacked by a stranger. I wasn't raped. I was strangled, and left for dead.

Instead of getting help, I was shocked, angry, felt betrayed by my mother, existed in survival mode, and ran as far away from my hometown in Arizona as I could get, which happened to be Louisiana. Shortly thereafter, I met the man who'd be my husband, and 10 months after I was attacked, we married.

Instead of grieving and healing, I dove into being his wife, raising our family, and burying the pain of my past, but that kind of pain cannot be denied. When suppressed pain can't find a direct path to the surface, it leaks out sideways.

It wasn't all sharp rocks and thorns and thistles. Not only did I get lucky in the grandmother, sister, and brother departments but also in the husband, children, and grandchildren departments too! My husband says, when we met, we were two lost souls that God brought together to love and heal each other, and he is absolutely correct. He made me feel safe and protected and cherished and loved, and 36 years, three children, five grandchildren, one divorce, and two marriages (to each other) later, I still feel the same way. He is my rock. The gift from the Universe that saved me, and I, him.

You know when you hit junior high school and you start thinking seriously about what you want to be when you grow up? Doctor, lawyer, teacher, engineer, president, stewardess, or actress? The possibilities are breathtakingly limitless. Me? I wanted to be a mother. Certainly a better mother than the one I had. In fact, I was going to be such a fabulous mother that I'd show her what she missed out on by being such a shitty one.

I was going to be super mom, super wife, super career woman, and started with the best of intentions. When it was just me, my husband, and our first son, it was easy. My messy, chaotic childhood and traumatic past seemed so far away, and our home was relatively tidy, clutter free, and full of love.

It wasn't until our second son came along that the demands of being a wife and working mother of two rambunctious little boys began to overwhelm me to the point that the bed didn't get made until just before we crawled into it at night, and dishes and laundry began to pile up.

By the time my sweet baby girl was born, the joy of a made bed wasn't even a whisper at the back of my mind anymore.

Sure, there were a couple of traumatic things that happened to me as a young woman, but I'd been able to successfully bury them and move on. Certainly one thing (trauma) had nothing to do with the other (clutter), right? Or maybe it did, but that wasn't a leap I could make until a couple of decades later.

Clutter is pernicious. It creeps up on you until you look around and your children are drowning in chaos, and you have no idea how it happened. Where was the tipping point?

Maybe that's what happened to my mother. It certainly gave me a greater sense of compassion for her.

As I struggled with the demands of being a wife and mother and an employee, I lost touch with the aspect of myself that found order liberating, and I slipped back into the chaos of clutter. That part of my mind that flourished in order slowly lost the battle against clutter. My mind let go of any hope of order, tuned out, and closed down.

I lived on the other side of the country from my family. Neither of my parents came to my wedding. Only my sister and her family were there. My mother and I spoke once every few years, saw each other once every five years or so. I lost touch with old friends and forgot my grandmothers' teachings.

Awakening

We lived that way for years. Not filthy, but not clean either. Clutter was a constant battle I often lost, and dishes and laundry were the bane of my existence.

Take laundry, for instance. The moment my kids were old enough to reach the washing machine, I taught them to sort, wash, dry, fold, and put away their own clothes. They were responsible for doing their own laundry from about 11 onward. As long as it didn't pile up in the laundry room, or bathroom, their clothes were their own business.

My oldest son and daughter are naturally organized, tidy people and kept their stuff that way. My husband and middle son? Not so much.

I am an avid reader – TV bores the hell out of me – always have been. There is nothing interesting to me in passively watching other people pretend to live interesting lives. In the evening, when my family settled in to watch a TV show, I'd head into another room to read a book.

On one such occasion, I read a book that changed my life and helped me put chaos and clutter into perspective, understand myself, and grasp the impact that my inability to deal with clutter had on my children.

I wish I could remember the book, or the author. I want to say it was Thich Nhat Hanh's *Living Buddha, Living Christ*, but couldn't swear to it. Also, it's been so long now that I'm not entirely sure the quote I'm about to share is 100% accurate, so I'll paraphrase, but here's the message I took away from it...

> "People who live in messy houses lead messy lives
> filled with chaotic emotions that swing wildly from one

extreme to another, with no ability to regulate them, much less get them under control long enough to create a plan, or see it through."

My life encapsulated in a sentence.

What I subjected my children to hit me in the gut so hard it took my breath away. While they didn't grow up in abject filth like I did at one point, they were certainly well acquainted with clutter, chaos, and disorganization.

I think this is what the Bible refers to when it talks about sins of the father...or mother, as the case may be. We infect our children with the emotional baggage of stumbling blocks we don't face, much less clean up.

There comes a moment of clarity in any mess where you wake up and realize something must change, and it can only be *you*. This mess I'd made "normal" for my children actually wasn't "normal" at all. It was baggage I'd inherited and was passing to the next generation. It wasn't even about me anymore, I had my children to think of too.

There was the house and family, with all its love, laughter, and joy, but also its clutter, chaos, and disorganization. There were the dirty dishes and baskets of unwashed (or clean, but unhung) clothes. And there was me. Out of all of them, the only variable that could change in that moment was me.

At first, I told myself I didn't know where to start, but that was just a habit of thought and not true. I loved crawling into a made bed. So, instead of waiting to make the bed right before I climbed in it, I got up and made it right then and promised myself I'd make my bed every morning, which I did for almost 12 years.

The smooth expanse of covers brings a special feeling of order and accomplishment to start my day, and this changed the tempo of the days that followed.

The next thing I did was tackle the linen closet.

Every house has a junk drawer, closet, or room. You know, that place where you shove the shit you don't want to deal with. The repository for the paint cans with leftover paint. The shoes with no match readily available, but you're still waiting for it to turn up one day. The odd assortment of hand tools, and wayward screws. That place you have to open slowly, and close quickly, least the contents fall out on top of your head.

My linen closet was the junk closet. There was no actual linen in the linen closet. Everything else, sure, but there was not a shred of linen to be found. So, I took everything out, cleaned the shelves, walls, and floor, then sorted the junk into piles: garage, storage, trash, donation, put away.

From that moment forward, the only thing that went into the linen closet was linen. Colorful towels, sheets, and blankets all neatly folded in orderly stacks. That's it.

I cannot tell you how much pleasure it gives me to open the linen closet and see the tidy rows of towels, sheets stored by sets, and blankets. It makes me giggle happily.

The feeling of order and spaciousness that filled me was so fulfilling, so empowering, I took on my bedroom closets next. I got rid of the hodgepodge of colored plastic hangers and replaced them with nice hangers. Black hangers for my husband, white hangers for me.

That's how it started. I wish I could say that' where my story ended, but it doesn't.

I'm not an efficiency expert – certainly no Martha Stewart – and I wasn't born with a clean gene. In the nature versus nurture debate, I'd have to say that nurture has had the most profound role in shaping who I am and setting my stumbling blocks in place. You can always tell the state of my mind by the state of my house. My grandmothers taught me how to piece my mind into a semblance of order, and I successfully maintained a clutter-free, tidy, organized home for almost 12 years.

That is, until my 31-year-old son, the sloppy one, moved back home two years ago and brought his pregnant girlfriend and her toddler with him. (There is a reason momma birds push their baby birds out of the nest. I'm just sayin'...) Yes, I've lapsed more than once, and had to clean it up. I'm in the process of doing that right now. The truth is, thanks to my grandmothers, I can do that.

While I love my granddaughters, and adore how their sweet giggles fill my home with innocent joy, I am not a fan of cleaning up after grown-ass adults who cannot seem to pick up after themselves, much less load or unload a freaking dishwasher.

It is stunning to me how quickly all my carefully organized systems collapsed into chaos and how difficult it's been to reclaim my equilibrium by establishing healthy boundaries.

I'd rather saw my own foot off than relive my childhood, or come face-to-face with the state I'd allowed my house to devolve into, or deal with the shame I have surrounding all of it.

And yet, here we are...

~ ~ ~ ~ ~

I've lived a life of struggle, mediocrity, and chaos punctuated by moments of brilliance and oodles of love and potential. In my soul, I knew I was created for a special purpose, we all are, but I was afraid I'd spent so much time trying to overcome my stumbling blocks that I wasn't even close to living my purpose.

Every stumbling block in your path, is an opportunity to learn lessons about yourself so you can evolve into the next best version of yourself.

My biggest gift, by far, is that I can find the good in anything. There is nothing that happens to you that you will not come out of better on the other side of it. Nothing.

Growing up messy as I did, a child of chaos and clutter, has given me so many blessings.

- No matter how big the mess, I can create order from chaos.
- I have come to the profound understanding that my mind creates my environment, and my environment creates my mind.
  - It doesn't matter which one I clean up first because the other will follow.

- It's easier to start with your environment because it doesn't lie like your ego does.

I know what it is to bury pain and fear. I know what it is to drown myself in layers of fat and clutter to hide from the world for decades. I know what it is to dig it all up, clean it all up, and to forgive – to find joy, peace, release, and glorious freedom.

And so can you.

Chapter 3 – Messy Bed, Messy Head

"If you quit on the process, you
are quitting on the results."
~Idowu Koyenikan

Chapter 3, and you're still with me?! Give yourself a high-five, pat yourself on the back, or go look in a mirror and tell your reflection how amazing you are! Most people who pick up a self-help book rarely make it past the first chapter because personal growth and development isn't for wussies.

The simple fact is this: There is no "easy way" to fully ripen and evolve into the magnificent Being you were Created to be! You have to be willing to walk through the garbage that keeps you from being who you want to be, and, let's face it, that shit is rotten and stinks!

(Better make that two high-fives!)

Where does clutter come from? The short answer is: you. (I may make you squirm uncomfortably from time to time, but I'll never lie to you.)

How to clean it up? I am a Life Coach and Transformation Strategist who specializes is helping my clients literally change their identity. You can go from smoker to non-smoker – a person who would never even consider picking up a cigarette to deal with stress – even if you've been a pack a day smoker for two decades. You can also go from drowning in messiness, chaos, and clutter, to a person who'd never consider leaving their bedroom without making their bed. Who you want to be is totally possible because who you were created to be lives within you. I'll show you how to peel back the layers of *stuff* that keeps you from experiencing your magnificence.

In working with my coaching clients, I created a process to cleaning things up, and believe it or not, it doesn't start with picking up the trash. It starts with looking at *why* the trash is there in the first place. Being willing to examine the trash objectively. Then you'll pick it up, see what baggage comes with it, and explore that too.

Human growth is messy. Beautiful, but messy. Painful, but necessary. Evolving from messy to orderly is a process, not an epiphany, and, in this book, I'll walk you through the journey I take my clients on to help them dig up, clean up, and release the things that clutter their lives.

The process flows like this...

Step 1 – Write Your Story

As the name of this step implies, first things first, you write out your story. Sunlight truly is the best disinfectant because the insight you'll gain into who you are, what formed your beliefs and habits, and why you do the wonky things you do will become crystal clear.

I learned so much invaluable information about myself in writing Chapter 2 that, from this point forward in my life coaching practice, I'll have all my clients write out their clutter history as the very first exercise.

It's such a powerful exercise, you just might blow your own mind, and in Chapter 4 of this book I'll walk you through the process of exploring your own history with messiness!

Seriously, digging into the past is a great way to blow out the cobwebs and bring repressed emotional baggage to the surface. Be sure to have a box of Kleenex handy, and be willing to feel the feels that arise fully.

Step 2 – Create A Compelling Vision

Why create a vision? To create momentum and give you a "Why" that will move you to action.

I know all you want is for your house to be clean, tidy, and organized – and to stay that way – so you won't feel embarrassed to invite someone over, or so your kids won't be mortified to have their friends see the inside of their house. But when you've been clean-averse for most of your life, the word "clean" is not enough to move you to action. (If it were, your house would be super shiny and spotless, but it isn't, now is it?)

In fact, it may even become so overwhelming that you abandon your cleaning, decluttering, and organizing project and run for the hills. You definitely don't want that!

Do you even know what you like? I'm not talking about the awesome home transformations you see on HGTV – we can all agree they're breathtaking – but what makes YOU feel at ease and at peace? It's important to understand *that* before you begin to overhaul your house, and I'll walk you through a couple of exercises designed to help you zero in on what aesthetic elicits a feeling of *HOME* for you.

You need a vision of where you want to go before you can create a map to get you there, so, in Chapter 5, I'll walk you through getting a clear vision of what you like, what you find aesthetically pleasing, and help you get a deep sense of what the word "home" feels like to you.

Step 3 – Keep Your Promises

Trust is earned. Self-trust is the most valuable, vulnerable, and fragile of all.

- How many times have you started something but not finished it?
- How many times have you tried to get a handle on your messy house only to give up in despair when the sheer magnitude of the task loomed before you?
- How many projects have you started on Monday, only to give up on by Tuesday or Wednesday, then shrugged them off as unimportant when the discomfort of change became too much to bear?

Every time you choose to walk toward your goal, a budding seed of accomplishment gets nurtured inside you. Every time you break a promise to yourself and turn away from your heart's desire, you deny that tiny seed nourishment and erode your own self-trust.

Newton's Third Law of Motion states: Every action has an equal and opposite reaction. Everything you do has a consequence. Everything has a price and a reward which is commensurate with your *actions*.

Creating a strong foundation of wellness begins with self-trust. In fact, you can gain no ground in any area of personal development until you trust yourself to keep your promises to yourself. Not by taking on some behemoth task, but by trusting yourself to do *today* what you say you are going to do.

As part of creating self-trust, you'll need to create a map/plan to get you where you want to go.

Let's say you get in your car in San Francisco heading toward New York City. Do you think you could actually get there without a map, or GPS, to at least point you in the right direction? Unless you're one of those fortunate people with a homing pigeon-like sense of direction, I'm going to go out on a ledge and guess: probably not!

Well, the same is true of any endeavor where you may know the goal, or destination, but have no clue how to get there. Cleaning, decluttering, and organizing your house is no different.

In Chapter 6, you shore up that foundation of self-trust so you can build upon it by making promises to yourself, and scheduling them on the calendar. You'll take the compelling vision of the home you want to raise your family in, and make a map/plan to get you to your destination.

Step 4 – Make Your Bed

Once you've bolstered your foundation of self-trust, and drawn yourself a map of where you want to go; in Chapter 7 it's time to put things into action. Not in huge, overwhelming tasks, but by breaking them down into bite-size chunks that are completely doable.

You're rebuilding self-trust, after all, so you'll want to start small, and making your bed is a good place to start.

The simple act of making your bed allows you to start the day with a win. Permit yourself to take a sense of pride in the smooth covers, and find joy in the beautiful, clutter-free oasis that is your bed.

You made your bed? Wahoooo! Celebrate the feeling of accomplishment. Girl, you deserve it! It won't be long before you're buying a fancy pillow or two, just to make it look prettier, and attending to the nightstand...and organizing the dresser...and buying matching hangers for the closet...

Also, the simple action of making your bed - creating order - sets in motion a chain reaction of neuropeptides in your brain and body that begin the task of creating order in your mind.

Seriously.

Neuroscience has shown us that the brain, what we once thought to be rigid and hard-wired, is actually plastic, malleable, and moldable at virtually any age. My brilliant proofreader, Sarah, also pointed out that science used to believe that the ability to create new neurons (neurogenesis) was only possible for children, but have now proved that it is possible for adults to create brand-spanking new neurons too.

That deserves a second WAHOOOOO in all caps!!!

Step 5 – Notice Your Thoughts

Once you get your vision, re-establish self-trust, make your plan, and take action, all the reasons you didn't do it in the first place will bubble up to the surface.

It may feel uncomfortable, and confusing, but, my dear, you are sitting on a goldmine for personal development that goes way, way, WAY beyond just cleaning your messy house! (Can I get a WAHOOOO???)

Notice your thoughts. Write them down. These are gems on your path that will open the door to your transformation from messy housekeeper to clean, clutter-free, organized, creative dynamo! (No hyperbole!)

And here's why...

According to Brooke Castillo's magnificent book *Self Coaching 101*, "your thoughts create your feelings, your feelings drive your actions, your actions dictate your results, and your results will ALWAYS prove your original thought."

You MUST prove yourself right. It is a biological imperative. Not only that, the quality of your thoughts is limited to your subconscious beliefs.

You could spend years in therapy hoping all your subconscious beliefs will eventually drift to the surface so you can evaluate and process them, or you can invite them to the surface by taking the very actions that you've avoided to keep them repressed.

Let's face it, your environment is merely a reflection of your interior. Paying attention to the thoughts and feelings that drive your actions and dictate your results will put you at a distinct advantage by knowing what the hell they actually are.

When you pay attention to your thoughts, you open the door to changing your fundamental beliefs.

Trust me, love, it's a win-win, and I'll show you how in Chapter 8!

Step 6 – Get Leverage On Yourself

1. What are you getting out of living in a messy house?
2. What is it costing you and your family?

These two questions are the carrot and the stick we'll use to change the beliefs that govern your behavior.

If you want to make a permanent change to your behavior, you must get leverage on yourself. Be willing to explore why you do what you do, and why you've done what you've done, with an open heart and mind filled with curiosity, acceptance, and compassion.

Love, acceptance, curiosity, and compassion form the foundation of wellness and provide the key to lasting transformation. But first, you need to blow out the cobwebs! To do that, you'll need to stir up a little pain because, as Tony Robbins says in his coaching programs Personal Power II, Get The Edge, and in every book he's ever written, or in any seminar he's ever given, "You will do more to avoid pain than you will ever do to gain pleasure."

Look, you're a fabulous person with a few bad habits, but habits can be changed. Finger-pointing, drama, and condemnation are useless endeavors that only ensure you'll feel worse about yourself as you continue the undesired behavior.

Pain, used consciously and intelligently, can drive the impetus to change, but you want to avoid getting stuck in a place of judgment and condemnation.

There is a huge difference between blame and responsibility. There is an even bigger difference between having habits that don't serve you, and believing your habits are your identity.

Taking responsibility from a place of love and self-compassion means being willing to explore where you've erred so you can free yourself from the things that no longer serve you.

In Chapter 9, I'll show you how to use pain and pleasure intelligently to arrive at a place of peace, understanding, and love.

Step 7 – A Place For Everything

In Chapter 10 you're going to finally, finally, FINALLY understand how and why clutter accumulates, and, best of all, how to put an end to it.

Having a place for everything is essential to a well-organized home. Things that do not have a place where they belong are shiftless, aimless and bring that shiftless, aimless, disorganizing energy into your home.

It's a good thing you learned the importance of noticing your thoughts in Chapter 8 because it is a vital skill that will come in super duper handy in this step. There's a part of you that will balk at getting rid of all the junk you've been hoarding. Thoughts will surface like, "but what if I need that 15-year old Nokia charger for something in the future?!" and you've now got a tool to deal with that psychic non-sense!

When I started cleaning, decluttering, and organizing my house, I started by cleaning one room and moving everything in it to another room, which made that other room look like it'd been struck by a natural disaster.

Turns out, I just moved piles of junk around from place to place, and, by the time I felt like I'd gained ground, the room I started with was trashed again. So frustrating!

Sound familiar?

I fought the battle with chaos and clutter for years until I learned quite recently to give all my possessions a home. In this step, I'll walk you through an exercise to create order and clarity in your house by assigning a home to the things you love, and getting rid of anything that doesn't spark peace, joy, and contentment within you.

Step 8 – What's Missing?

Self-discipline was a positive character trait I'd never bothered to cultivate within myself until I saw how the lack of it kept me small, even when I knew in my soul I was capable of great things.

What holds you back? Is it self-discipline, or self-honesty, or something else? In Chapter 11, I'll show you how to challenge yourself to take what was once a flaw, and transform yourself into the creative dynamo you know you were created to be!

Step 9 – Explore Your Mindset

#1 secret of the Universe: Now that you've got your vision, plan, and action set in motion, you'll face inevitable stumbling blocks.

Consider the possibility that these stumbling blocks are gifts from the Universe. Really, I swear they are!

Two challenges you're sure to run into when you first clean, declutter, and organize your home are: 1) living with slobs, and 2) your own mindset.

Face it, you may live with slobs, but they're slobs you've trained, so you'll have to take responsibility for that and untrain them. If your children are small, they'll balk at first, but young children are easily retrained and soon won't remember their formerly slobbish ways. Older children are more of a challenge, and I'll show you how to set appropriate boundaries with them.

The biggest struggle you'll face, by far, is your own mindset. In Chapter 12, I'll show you how your mind works, the purpose of each aspect of your mind, how habits are formed, why you need them, and, better yet, how to change those pesky habits that simply don't serve you, or your family.

Why do you need to know how your mind works? Once you understand how your mind works, how all the components fit together, you can change anything. Anything at all. Even your very identity.

Work these steps, and you'll be set to clean up your home, declutter your thought process, and change the quality your life, and the lives of your children, for the better in almost every way.

Any decluttering program will help you clean your house, and that is a beautiful, wonderful thing. *Messy Bed, Messy Head*, however, endeavors to get to the source of the clutter in the first place, and clean that up, so messiness is no longer an issue for you. *Messy Bed, Messy Head* is for those who want to go deeper than figuring out a way to do the dishes and put away the laundry to release themselves from mediocrity, and reach for the spark of divinity that lives within each one of us.

I get you completely. You want to stop being embarrassed by your house. You want a home filled with love and laughter and family and friends. You want your children to feel safe, protected, and not be riddled with the shame and embarrassment of living in a dirty house.

Close your eyes and imagine you're the type of woman who is a clean, clutter-free, and organized creative dynamo! A woman who'd never allow her home to become messy because it isn't in her nature to do so. A woman who takes pride in her home, her family, and, most importantly, herself. The vision tugs at your heart because it is who you really are.

The seed of who you are, who you were born to be before the world shaped and molded you with its messiness, lives deep in your heart, or in the pit of your gut. Not your head. And the path to who you really are is your intuition. Your inner guide. Your inner truth.

When you live in a messy house, you want to "change who you are," but when you clean, declutter, and organize your home, you have an opportunity to peel away the barriers the outer world foisted upon you, strip away the superfluous, and reveal your true identity.

Over the course of my lifetime, I've changed my identity several times. I went from being a smoker to a non-smoker; from sloppy to tidy; from angry, sad and miserable to happy, grateful, and content; and from a woman too petrified to open her mouth in public to a Distinguished Toastmaster and paid public speaker. Changing your identity is absolutely possible.

Through this process, I'm going to show you how to shed the illusions that produce messiness (and can never produce anything but) and embrace the woman you dream of being. The woman who would never allow her home to get out of hand lives deep inside you. You picked up this book because she's crying for your attention. I'll show you how to set her free...

Messy Bed, Messy Head (MBMH) Housekeeping

To transform your home into the clean, inviting safe haven you dream of, you've got to take action and put in the work required to complete the transformation. It's not enough to just read the book, you're going to have to get your hands dirty. Thoughts create the impetus to transform, but action takes the thought and makes it a reality.

To effectively work this program, and successfully transform your house into a warm, inviting home, there are three things that are non-negotiable must-haves:

1. A journal/workbook
2. A daily planner/calendar
3. The heart of an explorer

Transformation isn't an overnight event. As I say over and over again, it is a process, not an epiphany. I created this program to take my life coaching clients through this material over the course of 8 weeks. As such, I recommend you do this slowly – one chapter a week – to really give yourself time to work the exercises, apply the material, and integrate the lessons into your life. If you need more than a week, by all means, take two, but whatever you do, don't short-change yourself by rushing this process.

You can do this program and transform your home, and your life, by following the steps in this book, and doing the exercises, but if you want a coach to work with you on a deeper level, I've got your back. I coach this program online, and would love to have you join us. Consider this an open invitation to apply for my Messy Bed, Messy Head coaching program to work with me directly. https://www.cindylcooley.com/

Not sure if life coaching is right for you?

Feel free to go to my website to sign-up for a free mini-session. https://www.cindylcooley.com/work-with-me/

The MBMH program is not a passive process. As you might've guessed, there is a fair bit of writing associated with this process, so, to help you along, I created a free workbook with all the prompts and plenty of space to journal and write. Just go to my website https://www.cindylcooley.com/workbook/ to download it before you get started.

As for your daily planner/calendar, there is only one criteria: You MUST have a daily timeline breakdown so you can chunk your time. I wish planners had 15-minute increment breakdowns, but they don't. (At least, I've never run across one.) 30 minutes is the best you're going to get, so we'll make it work.

- Got your workbook?
- Got your planner?
- Ready to explore?!

Let's get to work!

Chapter 4 – Write Your Story

"There is surrendering to your story,
and then a knowing that
you don't have to stay in your story."
~Colette Baron-Reid

This is the smallest chapter in this book – you're welcome! – but it's also potentially the most powerful.

Before you lift a finger to clean your house, it's imperative to revisit your history to gain a better understanding of who you are, and how you evolved, so you can develop a super clear vision of what you want. Not just an "oh, that's pretty...or nice," but a profound sense of what triggers the ease, safety, and sense of belonging that transforms a house into a *home*. Not just for you, but for your children, your partner, your family, and friends.

Your Clutter Story

In her fabulous book *Wishcraft: How To Get What You Really Want*, Barbara Sher says the first step to getting what you want is to bring up all the old energy that prevents you from getting what you want in the first place. She has her readers write out all the reasons they can't have what they want. She says to kvetch, wail, and bemoan the universe for the horrors you've endured because until you look at those thoughts that hold you back in the light of day they will ALWAYS hold you back.

Sunlight truly is the best disinfectant because, after all these years, until I wrote Chapter 2, "Growing Up Messy," and really dove into and examined my experience with chaos and clutter in my formative years, I had no idea what I liked, why I liked it, or why I did the things I've done and continue to do. It never occurred to me to revisit my childhood with this laser-like focus on what it was like to grow up messy.

I learned so much invaluable information about myself in writing that chapter that, from this point forward in my life coaching practice, I'll have all my clients write out their history with their particular stumbling block as the very first exercise.

Here's an example of what I discovered about myself: I'm weird in that I love to move. Most people hate it, but not me. My husband is an engineer, and over the past 36 years, we've moved more than 25 times and lived in ten states (some states multiple times) and two countries. Every time we've moved, I've researched the area we're going to (thank you, internet) to find out what's fun to do.

I love to go to new places, meet new people, and do new things, but I never knew why until I wrote my story out. My mother used to say it's because I've got a gypsy's soul, but after writing my story, I understand it's because, when I was a child, after our house burned down, I made a powerful neuroassociation—that the hope, joy, and anticipation of empty, uncluttered living spaces was connected to moving to new houses.

That would translate into me loving to move as an adult? Who knew?! Certainly not I, until I brought it up and looked at it.

In the very first exercise, I want you to take a deep-dive as you revisit and write your history/struggle with clutter. Own everything. Write all of it out. Hold nothing back.

Before you begin, make sure you have a box of tissues within easy reach, have your favorite beverage on hand, go potty, turn your ringer off, and block out at least an hour, if not two, with no kids, or interruptions of any kind, so you don't have to get up or break the energetic flow of the exercise.

If you're like most people, you haven't done a deep-dive on your childhood clutter in decades, if ever. If you've ever wondered why you do what you do, you're likely to discover the roots of it here.

Your feelings may start to flow, and it's important to just let them ebb and flow of their own accord. Don't try to capture a particular feeling, don't try to hold on to it, and whatever you do, don't push any feelings away.

Don't hold anything back, don't filter what you write, and for goodness sake, don't edit it! Just write!

But – and here's the kicker – do it all with a sense of curiosity and compassion.

Sleep on this for a day or two – certainly overnight at least – and just see what bubbles up to the surface. Be sure to capture what surfaces, as well as your takeaways.

Pull out your workbook, aaannnndddd, GO...

Chapter 5 – Create A Compelling Vision

"He who has a why to live can bear almost any how."
~Friedrich Nietzsche

Now that you're starting to have an idea of *why* you do what you do, it's time to get a sense of what you like, what you find aesthetically pleasing, what elicits that profound sense of ease, safety, and belonging that will transform your house into a home your children will be proud to invite their friends over to.

Your husband, your children, your family and friends take their cues from you. If you feel at ease in your home, they will feel at ease too. If you feel safe in your home, they will also feel safe. If you are in a state of chaos, they will live in a state of chaos as well.

When it comes to knowing what makes a house feel like a home, most of us have no clue what triggers that deeper sense of ease, safety, and belonging that transforms a house into a home.

Can you picture your home as a clean, welcoming, inviting space? Do you know what you like? What appeals to you? Most of us inherit our sense of style from our mothers, our friends' mothers, or our grandmothers, aunties, and friends, but have you ever taken the time to really know what *moves* you emotionally? Have you ever sat with the colors you typically surround yourself with to see how your body responds to them?

Binge on Porn

Girl, get your mind out of the gutter! In the Cindy-verse, "porn" is merely visual or written material designed to elicit interest or arousal. There's food porn, earth porn, word porn, minimalist porn, organizational porn, and, of course, porn porn, but in reality, the options are limitless. In this case, we're talking House Porn! (I truly dig House Porn!)

Spend an afternoon at Barnes & Noble, your local library, or browse online perusing house porn. I adore going to B&N because they have those big, comfy chairs there. I invite you to curl up with the magazines and books that speak to you, and take note of the emotions that well up inside you. (Don't forget to bring your journal with you. You'll need it.)

- What colors speak to you?
    - Where do you feel it in your body?
- What colors repel you?
    - Where do you feel THAT in your body?
- What aesthetic gives you a sense of peace?
- What aesthetic makes you feel scattered?

Browse real estate websites, and look at high-end houses in the place you would LOVE to live. Watch for the architectural elements and design styles that make you gasp with awe and giggle happily.

Make note of the house porn you keep coming back to, sure, but also look deeply at the elements and styles you have a strong negative response to, too. When your emotions speak to you, whether supposedly positive or negative, there is a message for you in that. It's your job to ferret out what that means, and it's not always what seems obvious to your ego. (In Chapter 12 I go into detail about the ego, and how it seeks to protect you, so it will most likely posit something unfamiliar as potentially negative, or threatening, until you consciously determine it is not.)

Because I am my best resource/reference, let me share this example with you...

I'd inherited a "country" aesthetic from my sister and 80s culture, which I never questioned. It was the style I was most exposed to, so I never thought much about it.

I've always loved to peruse *Architectural Digest*, *Good Housekeeping*, and the multitude of lifestyle magazines over the years, but turned my nose up at the stark minimalist and modern designs. In fact, those rather stark designs created a stronger, albeit negative, emotional response within me than the "country cottage" look ever did.

Although my brain screamed "nooooo" at the very thought of the cold, clinical whiteness of the modern aesthetic, something deeper within me kept coming back to it.

I thought I'd rather die than have white walls, so I painted the rooms in my house every color of the rainbow. I went for the dark, bold colors because they felt warm and comforting, and I loved them so much. But, at some point, living with those dark colors began to feel heavy and burdensome. Like I was living in a cave that eventually collapsed and trapped me inside. I began to feel claustrophobic to the point that, now, I find myself longing for lightness, simplicity, and minimalism.

Turns out, the deep emotional response to the simplicity and elegance of modern design was simply my deeper knowing bringing them to my attention, but I was so out of tune with my intuition that I interpreted these feelings as negative because they were unfamiliar.

~~~~~

Visualization For Non-Visualizers

"Visualize this thing that you want. See it, feel it, believe in it.
Make your mental blueprint, and begin to build."
~Robert Collier

Now that you know your story, understand why you do what you do, and have a sense of what you like and don't like, it's time to visualize the home you want to create for your family.

Creating a compelling vision for your home starts, quite literally, with visualization.

The next exercise is all about cementing the vision BEFORE you create it.

You may be wondering, "But how do I visualize?"

The short answer is, create a picture in your mind, and make it so real that you can see it, feel it, touch it, taste it. But how? There isn't a single way.

There is no "right" way to visualize. There is only *your* way.

Many, many of you can paint a mental picture in your mind's eye of what you want, and I think that is AWESOME! I'm so happy for you. But I am not Picasso and cannot paint a picture in my mind to save my soul. Come to find out, I am not alone.

For every two people who are mental visualizers, five of you are NOT.

If you are one of the majority who simply can't do it, I've got great news for you...

Rather than reinvent the wheel, I'd love to share this article I wrote for TUT.com a couple of years ago...

Manifestation for Non-Visualizers

Are you frustrated because you've tried, and tried, and tried to visualize what you want to manifest, but you just don't "SEE" things? You're not alone!

Fear that you'll never be able to manifest what you want because you can't visualize it? Yes, you can!

There is another way to visualize anything you'd like to manifest without struggling to project an image that just won't come.

It starts with YOU!

As a non-visualizer myself, I'll show you how I discovered how to use my personal creative outlet to manifest the things I want in my life, and I'll show you how you can too!

I used to get so frustrated trying to "visualize," that all I wound up manifesting in my life was frustration – heaps of it, in fact – until, one day, I finally gave up and took my problem to the Universe in prayer and meditation, then let it go.

A few weeks later, I had a dream: I sat at an ornate desk, writing on parchment with a vibrant peacock quill. As I wrote the word "HORSE," a powerful black stallion leapt off the page. I wrote the word "CASTLE," and a palace worthy of the greatest fairytale materialized around me.

The next morning, I woke up feeling breathless and excited!

The message was very clear: I am a writer, so write! My brain is already hardwired to create pictures with words. That's how I "SEE." It only makes sense that, if I want to manifest something specific, I should utilize how my brain *actually* works, and WRITE my visualizations.

Mind. Blown.

Your Gorgeous Brain

Flick the switch a light is wired to, and the light comes on. Flick a different switch hoping it will affect that same light? You get nothing.

Think of your brain like the wiring of a house. Over the course of your lifetime, your thoughts, words, and actions have wired/trained your mind to behave in a specific way. (Those are called neuropathways.)

Now, think of visualizing as flicking a light switch. You can try to visualize somebody else's way, but if your neuropathways aren't wired to that particular switch, you can toggle the switch all you want, but it will never power the light you want lit.

Tap Into Your Creative Outlet

How do you express yourself?

Are you a painter? Writer? Dancer? Quilter? Chef? Gardener? Photographer? The list is endless, and it makes no difference which one you are. The only requirement is that it has to be the conduit for YOUR creative flow.

What is YOUR creative outlet? You don't have to be an artist. What do you do that makes you FEEL heard, seen, expressed, and/or complete?

Put yourself in that creative state by engaging in that activity, and go to town with your creative visualizations!

Paint your visualizations, if you're a painter. Write your visualizations, if you're a writer. Dance, and feel your dreams flood every cell of your body as you do so, if you're a dancer.

Harness the Creative Power of Emotion

Creativity is the outpouring of emotion manifested into physical form, and it is POWERFUL.

When you're engaged in creative visualization to manifest what you want to bring into fruition, it's important not to force your emotions to be "happy" while you're in the creative state. Let your feelings be whatever they are, and allow them to well and ebb and flow freely. Creativity isn't always a happy, joyful experience. Sometimes it's frustrating, and that's perfectly okay.

Fill your body full of creative energy, and incorporate whatever it is you want to manifest into that.

Since I started writing my visualizations a few years ago, my ability to draw to myself that which I ask for is quite staggering!

I watched a wonderful webinar on a course I would love, love, LOVE to take, but I didn't have $400 cash on hand for the full course, so I didn't think twice about it. Two days later, they sent me the replay of the webinar, and I watched it again, taking careful notes.

The act of incorporating the creative energy of my writing – along with my strong desire to experience the material being presented, and adding it to the creative energy of taking (and then retaking) the class – sent a powerful message to the Universe that I desired the class.

The next day, I met with my business coach and shared with her how awesome the webinar was, but I didn't tell her how much I wanted to take the class.

She said, "You know, Cindy, I think I bought that class last year but forgot about it."

After checking her e-mail – and finding that she had, indeed, purchased the class but never did anything with it – she gifted me the entire $400 class on the spot!

Things like that happen often in my life, which never happened before I discovered the joy of working with my creative outlet instead of fighting to supplant it.

What a magnificent gift your brain is! Learn how to harness its creative energy, and you can use it to fuel your dreams. Try to make it zig when it's wired to zag, and you'll have a constant struggle on your hands.

Use your brain – how it is currently wired to be the conduit for your creative energy – as your means of visualization, and I can guarantee you the quality, and quantity, of your manifestations will increase dramatically!

This may sound a bit "woo woo" to you, but your life is an amalgamation of the thoughts you choose to think, the emotions you create, and the actions you take on a regular basis. It begins with thoughts, so, as TUT.com's creator Mike Dooley's tagline says, "Thoughts become things. Choose the good ones."

If all you focus on is the mess you're currently living in, that is all you'll create.

You deserve a home that welcomes you the moment you step through the door, and so do your children and husband. Getting a clear vision of the home you want to create for your family is the starting point for everything you will build from this point forward.

Exercise: Use Your Creative Outlet to "Visualize"

The questions below are just prompts to open your thought

process, or you can discard them altogether. There are no right or wrong answers here. The important thing is to get a sense of what you like on a deeper level.

And, trust me, there is ALWAYS a deeper level. There is your head (ego), which is the voice that chatters non-stop and is apt to lead you on a merry chase. There is your heart, which feels beneath the surface and powers your desires. And finally, there is your gut – that deeper level of "knowing" – which is often the seat of your intuition. (I say "often" because many people experience their intuition in their heart, but mine is most definitely in my gut.)

Experience your home now. Not as it is, but as you'd love it to be, and, as you do so, you lay the foundation for the home you'll create for your family.

Use all the creative avenues open to you to create that visual impression of "home" so you'll have the direction in which to move as you clean, declutter, and organize your home.

Take your time, as much time as you need, and don't rush through this.

Some suggestions for this creative exercise:
- Create a vision board with all the beautiful pictures that elicit an emotional response within you. (If you make a vision board, please put a picture of your family and yourself on it. I cannot tell you how many people create vision boards for their lives but forget to put themselves in the vision too!)
- Write a detailed description of your ideal home room by room.

- Paint a landscape-style portrait of each room as you want it to be.
- And, of course, if you're one of those fabulously fortunate visualizers, visualize away.

Sit in meditation for 2-3 minutes each morning, and each night before you go to bed, to embody the vision so that it compels you forward. Do this for a minimum of the remaining seven weeks of this program, and you will enlist the limitless power of your subconscious mind as a partner to help you create this reality.

Chapter 6 – Keep Your Promises

"The most important person to
keep a promise to is yourself."
~Anonymous

Welcome to Step 3 in the Messy Bed, Messy Head process! Woot woot! Like I said before, most people who pick up a book designed to make a difference in their lives, and help them move through the obstacles necessary to overcome a particular stumbling block, rarely get past the first chapter, much less the first step.

But not you! Nope, you made it through your skepticism and pessimism, and you're here! You deserve a second, WOOT WOOT!!!

In Step 3, you'll shore up that foundation of self-trust so you can build upon it by making and keeping promises to yourself. You'll take the compelling vision of the home you want to raise your family in, make a map/plan to get you to your destination, and put the tasks on the calendar so you'll actually do them.

Let's get started on Step 3 – Keep Your Promises...

Can You Trust Yourself?

Why is keeping the promises you make to yourself so important? No need to conk yourself over the head with an iron fist of judgment, or beat yourself up, but it's time for some tough self-love.

Everything in existence has a constructive aspect and a destructive aspect. If not tended to carefully, love can warp into obsession, and something as noble as service can be twisted into martyrdom. Honesty is no exception to the duality of existence. Honesty shines a light on truth and illuminates the darkness, whereas brutal honesty, the kind that tears you down and makes you feel worthless, is violent and abusive.

There is no place for brutality here. It's soooo not necessary. All exploration, whether of yourself, your family, your home, your community, or even your country, should be done with absolute respect for the wholeness and divineness of all. From the homeless person sleeping in a gutter to the super star, and every person you pass on the street was created from the same holy source as you. Every. Single. One.

I invite you to explore the following questions with a sense of curiosity and self-compassion, and ask that you answer these questions with unflinching honesty. (Unflinching self-honesty tempered with curiosity and compassion may seem mutually exclusive, but they're definitely not!) This is personal, private, and just between you and I. If you're really taking a deep-dive on this, it can get uncomfortable. Stay with the feelings. Write them down. Explore them. You are opening yourself up when you've been closed down, so it's only natural.

Please know that I hold sacred space for you as you delve into these questions and have absolute respect for your privacy, your experience of life, and your willingness to walk into the discomfort to get to what's real.

Now, time to break out your workbook...

1. How many times have you started something but not finished it?
    a. How does that make you feel about yourself?
2. How many times have you tried to get a handle on your messy house only to give up in despair when the sheer magnitude of the task loomed before you?
3. How many times have you looked at those dirty dishes in the sink, or the piles of laundry waiting to be sorted, washed, dried, and put away, and chose to ignore them instead?
    a. How does that make you feel about yourself?
4. How many diets, or projects, or goals have you started working toward on Monday, only to give up on them by Tuesday or Wednesday, as you shrugged it off as unimportant when the discomfort of change became too much to bear?
5. How many times have you disappointed yourself by giving up on your dream, or goal, or plan, then told yourself it didn't matter anyway, when, in reality, it did? It really, really did.

If those questions felt a bit uncomfortable, good! It means you're hitting emotional pay dirt.

Every time you choose to walk toward your goal, a budding seed of accomplishment gets nurtured inside you. Every time you break a promise to yourself and turn away from your heart's desire, you deny that tiny seed nourishment and erode your own self-trust.

Newton's Third Law of Motion states: Every action has an equal and opposite reaction. Everything has a price and a reward which is commensurate with your actions. The price of creating the habit of breaking promises to yourself is erosion of your fundamental self-trust; the reward is a life half-lived, which is filled with disappointment, despair, and disillusion that can turn into bitterness. The price of creating the habit of keeping promises to yourself is work, or, as my Grandma Kiddoo liked to call it, sweat equity or elbow-grease; the reward is authentic pride, optimism, satisfaction, and the ability to create anything you want in life. Anything.

Creating a strong foundation begins with self-honesty and self-trust. (I'll talk more about self-honesty in Chapter 11.) In fact, you can gain no ground until you trust yourself to keep your promises to yourself. Not by taking on some behemoth task, but by trusting yourself to do *today* what you said you were going to do, when you said you were going to do it. And then doing it *again* tomorrow, and the day after, and the day after that.

The best way I know of to create self-trust is to do what you tell yourself you'll do. Period.

Bonus: Self-trust is also the basis of authentic confidence. (A topic for another book, but certainly worth an honorable mention here.)

Here is how I operated in the past. It may, or may not, sound familiar to you...

You're half-afraid someone is going to call child protective services on you because your house is so messy. You know you've got to clean it up, so you decide you're going to change your ways forever and clean your house from top to bottom. Visions of a sparkling clean home fill your mind's eye. Dishes are always done all the time, you make your children's beds every morning, vacuuming the carpet in pearls like June Cleaver, laundry never accumulates, and those dust bunnies living atop your picture frames and baseboards will find a new home! Sparkly rainbows shoot from your rooftop, and unicorns graze on your lawn.

Buuuuttttt then – even if you can't bring yourself to question the possibility that sparkly rainbows or unicorns *may* not exist – the reality of getting down on your hands and knees to scrub (what feels like) 84,000 feet of baseboards in your home kicks in, and the tediousness of everything else you must do to make it an actuality sinks in, as does overwhelm, anxiety, and depression, which are easier to deal with if you simply close your eyes and ignore the situation like you've done so, soooooo many times before. (Does that sound like the voice of experience? It should!)

Or, you get caught up in what Tony Robbins in his Get The Edge Program calls "the pressure cooker." This is when you feel the pressure to change that builds to the point that you HAVE to take action, so you do, then things improve, so you feel better. But once you feel better, you stop taking action. You drift along until the pressure to change starts to build again, and the cycle starts all over again.

Time to ditch the pressure cooker, and climb off of the emotional roller coaster!

You are not a failure! You are not weak! You are not a slob! You are not a pig! You are not a horrible wife and mother (if you were, you wouldn't torture yourself like this!). It's not because you were bullied, or because your mother was a terrible housekeeper! You, my beautiful friend, have disempowering habits. Period. And disempowering habits can be changed once you open your eyes to them, take responsibility for them, change your thinking, make a plan, and take action.

(More on habits – how they're formed, why we need them, and how to change them – in Chapter 12.)

Baby Steps And The Zone of Proximal Development

I know that sounds like the title to a Harry Potter-esque book, but it's not. It's actually the key to effective, permanent transformation. Read on, my beautiful friend...

The problem when it comes to changing your life is *you're taking on too much too soon*. It's as simple as that. Unless you're presented with a burning bush, or a lightning bolt delivered via the wrath of God, you will not "change your life" in one fell swoop.

It doesn't happen that way. Remember, it's a process, not an epiphany!

Unfortunately, we live in an instant-gratification society, where maturation is rushed, and growth and development are pooh-poohed as arbitrary, when, in fact, they are not negotiable. Try as you may, but you will not sit down at a piano and bang out Bach if you've never touched a piano key. Doesn't happen.

True growth is incremental. A baby does not come out of the womb walking, talking, and making good decisions. It's a process that takes time, and it cannot be rushed.

As I mentioned in Chapter 2, I have a crazy multi-generational home. There is my husband and I, our 31-year-old son, who is injured and cannot work at the moment, his fiancé, their two daughters, and my 78-year-old mother with dementia is coming for an extended visit with us in a couple of weeks, which should round things out nicely. (😵)

My sweet li'l granddaughter Emily Grace is 14 months old, and she lives in my home. I had the unspeakable joy of watching her birth. I've been an integral part of her daily life and have observed her development closely. She started tensing her body at her core, doing deep abdominal conditioning by three weeks after birth, which is the precursor to rolling over, sitting, crawling, walking, and eventually running and climbing on everything (including my bookcases, and the hearth when Pawpaw makes a fire.) Each phase of her development is predicated upon the success of the previous phase, and she could not move forward until that previous phase had been fully mastered.

You are no different, my dear. You do not stand outside of the laws of nature, and I'd like to bitch-slap the idiot who convinced you, and me, and everyone else otherwise. In fact, I think we've all been sold a bill of goods that has made us feel like things should be "easy," or there's something wrong if we encounter struggle; that we are "special and deserving" regardless of our behavior, but if we don't get what we want, we struggle needlessly with the perceived reality that we...sniff...aren't really "special" at all. It puts a terrible burden on people to *always* be happy and *always* feel special, which is actually useless in helping us obtain our full potential.

So, what exactly is the zone of proximal development (ZOPD)? Think of a bull's eye target with three concentric rings...

You, beautiful goddess, as you currently are, stand in the center. The goal you'd like to achieve, but currently do not have the skill to obtain – a clean home that is a welcoming oasis of clutter-freeness – stands in the outer ring. Between those concentric circles, in the place just beyond your current abilities, but where you could get to with proper guidance, lies the zone of proximal development.

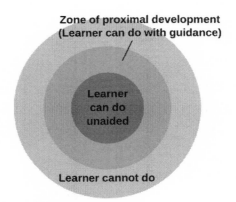

Image grabbed from Wikipedia

Start where you are, and build skill and confidence one tinsy, tiny baby step at a time. You won't be different tomorrow, or even next week, but within a year, step-by-step, your life will be completely transformed, and so will your children, your marriage, and your home. Work with a credible guide just beyond the edge of your comfort zone. That's where all your progress and growth are.

Why the zone of proximal development is important will become clear in the next step, but it's important to introduce it beforehand because you're going to create a map to your compelling vision, and it's important that you don't get bogged down in overwhelm.

Overwhelm = Paralyzation!

At this point, you've created a compelling vision, understand the importance of self-trust, and know the value of working within the zone of proximal development to create lasting change. Now it's time to make some decisions, create a plan, schedule tasks, and then work the plan.

Make a Decision

The word "decide" actually means *to cut off*. To make a true decision means that you cut yourself off from any other possibility. You've got your compelling vision, but do you want it enough to cut yourself off from the possibility of not having it?

I'm not going to spend a lot of time on this because there is no need to belabor the point. Do you choose to clean up the mess, regardless of the time it takes, or do you choose to wallow in it? There is power in decision. Profound, door-opening, Universe-changing, power.

Pull out your workbook, and let's get to work...

Brainstorm 10-Minute Tasks

You've got your vision and have made the decision that you're going to clean up the mess. I know you're either ready to get to work, or immediately regretting your decision to tidy. Both are perfectly normal, but if you're still reading this, it's because you've decided to put your house in order! Woot woot!

Before you put on those ratty old clothes you can throw away when you're done, roll up your sleeves, and get to work, you need to figure out what you're going to do. That's where brainstorming is invaluable.

A brainstorming session is exactly what it sounds like: You write down everything that comes into your mind about everything that needs to be done to clean your house WITHOUT filter.

I'm not a mind-mapper – and don't really understand the process enough to explain it – but if you are, by all means, go for it!

In this exercise, you're going to brainstorm a list of tasks that need to be done to clean up your house. But instead of sweeping categories like "laundry," I want to break things up into 10-minute tasks like this:

- Gathering the dirty clothes is a 10-minute task.
- Sorting laundry is a 10-minute task.
- Cycling clothes from the washer to the dryer and putting on another load of clothes to wash is a 10-minute task.
- Folding a basket of laundry is a 10-minute task.
- Sweeping the kitchen floor is a 10-minute task.
- Taking out the trash and putting a new trash bag in the

bin is a 10-minute task.

Got it? Don't stop to edit it. Just write!

Remember, if you haven't already downloaded the workbook, you can get it here: www.cindylcooley.com/workbook.

Got your workbook handy? Pull out your phone, and set the timer for 10 minutes. And GO...

All done? Now, asterisk the most important tasks. There are a number of things that "need" to be done, but where do you start? The short answer is: the thing that's been nagging at you the most. (Just don't start with making your bed because that is in the next chapter!)

Make a Plan

Rome wasn't built in a day, and, unless you have no children, husband, pets, family, friends, growling tummy, biological functions, or life to interrupt your time, your home won't be cleaned in a day either. But, if you work in chunks of three to five 10-minute tasks a day, it can be spic and span in just a few short weeks.

We'll discuss maintenance and the importance of daily rituals in Chapter 12. But for now, break out your calendar.

Calendaring

If you often find yourself drifting through life, spinning your wheels, and not really going anywhere - I used to tell myself it was because I wanted to be spontaneous – it's because you don't keep a daily calendar.

If you love to set goals but don't actually accomplish them, it's because you don't keep a daily calendar.

Poor time management is, without a doubt, the number one reason why I accomplished very little until after the age of 52, when I started keeping a calendar for the first time in my life. (It's *never* too late to start a new habit!)

I had huge dreams that came to nothing but bitterness and disillusionment until I forced myself to buy a freaking planner, and learned how to budget my time effectively. It wasn't growing up with a hoarder-esque mother, or the trauma of assault that went untreated. No, it was the lack of keeping a disciplined calendar that kept my life spinning into nowhere.

If you don't have a daily calendar, you need to go buy one immediately. Barnes & Noble carry them, so do Office Depot, Wal-Mart, and Target, not to mention Amazon has a plethora of planners. Make sure you get a DAILY planner with time you can block off and a place for tasks. (Mine has room for daily gratitude, tasks, and goals so I can keep them top of mind at all times.)

If you've got one but don't really use it, break it out and dust it off.

Go ahead, I'll wait...

Now that you've got your calendar, take your brainstorming list and schedule one 10-minute task for tomorrow. Just one task. (Remember, it can't be making your bed because that is task 2 in the next chapter/week!)

Why just one task? Because your calendar is more important than the tasks right now.

ONLY PUT THINGS ON YOUR CALENDAR THAT YOU WILL ACTUALLY DO!!!

(I cannot stress that enough. Indeed, if I could put dancing pandas, or a spotlight around this sentence to signify its importance, I would. Obviously, I cannot, so the bold, all caps, underlined, italicized, centered text with multiple exclamation marks will have to do, but you get my point...)

Remember, love, you're building self-trust. Budgeting your time by putting things on your calendar is important. But doing what you say you're going to do is the MOST important thing right now.

What is the one thing that's nagging at you? Schedule that tomorrow, and do it. No matter what. It may feel like the Universe is conspiring to make the 10-minute task you scheduled at a specific time impossible to follow through on, but it's not. (That's your ego throwing up roadblocks, but we'll get to that in Chapter 12.) This is where the proverbial rubber meets the proverbial road.

You're not interested in speed. You're interested in the *doable*.

There is plenty of time to develop daily rituals around maintaining your home – we'll certainly get to those later – but for now, take a week, one whole week, to schedule *ONE* task a day. Do that task – no excuses, no matter what – and allow yourself to feel a sense of authentic pride and accomplishment when you're done!

My beautiful friend, pat yourself on the back, and take pleasure in the fact that you made a promise to yourself and followed through.

Next week, you're going to put two 10-minute tasks on your calendar per day, and the week after that, you'll do three 10-minute tasks a day. Make sure you do them – no excuses, no matter what – and allow yourself to feel a sense of authentic pride and accomplishment when you're done. Generate the feeling that you're a Boss. A total badass Boss, at that!

When you feel tempted to postpone the 10-minute tasks you've put down on your calendar – and you most certainly WILL be tempted – stop and ask yourself, "How will I feel about myself if I *don't* keep my promise to myself? What future am I creating for myself, my children, and my husband by pretending that this one tiny broken promise doesn't matter?"

It's critically important to reward yourself with feeling good about what you've accomplished, and it's also important to call yourself out on your own bullshit. When you tell yourself that it doesn't matter, or it won't make a difference, or you'll do it next time, you are lying to yourself. It matters. It really, really does.

The snail's pace may chafe, but you're building new muscle here. Remember, you're in this for the long haul...

Chapter 7 – Make Your Bed

"Order is Heaven's first law."
~Alexander Pope, An Essay on Man
(1733-34), Epistle IV, line 49

This will be the second shortest chapter in this entire book – again, you're welcome – but perhaps most informative.

You've uncovered your history, created a compelling vision, broke it down into 10-minute tasks, put a one on your calendar last week, and did it faithfully. Now it's time to get busy and work on your tasks! Remember that 10-minute daily task you scheduled on your calendar in Chapter 6? Well, you're going to add one more thing to that - make your bed every morning.

A person with too much order in their lives can become rigid and unyielding and could use a little mess to loosen them up! But that's not your problem, now is it?

Having grown up in a messy house, and having raised my own children in a messy house for most of their formative years, I am familiar with the chaos a disordered mind can fabricate, and the web it spins can catch everyone you love in its destructive wake.

Why is that? It's because your exterior - all the things in your environment, which include your body, your home, your family, and your car - are a reflection of your mind, and your thought processes.

You bridge the gap between who you are now, and what you've produced in the world thus far by *changing your actions*.

We're going to go into thought-work in great detail in the next chapter, but for now, it is enough to understand that all you have to do is look around at the world you've created for yourself, and your family, to know the state of your mind.

A messy mind begets a messy home. You can go into therapy for years and hope that you find the issues that have held you back and will help you clean up the mess; or you can clean up the mess *first*, and all the reasons you've avoided doing it will bubble up to the surface.

What? I've said that before? Yes, yes I have – so glad you noticed – and I'll say it over and over again until you "know" the Truth of it because it is such powerful knowledge for anyone wishing to transform any area of their life!

Why does the military insist soldiers make their bed daily? The title of this book says it ALL: Messy Bed, Messy Mead! Making your bed each morning starts a chain reaction in your brain that is great for your mental health. Consider making your bed a gateway drug to other life-affirming, order-inducing habits.

Benefits of making your bed first thing every morning:
- You start the day with a feeling of accomplishment.
- The physical act of creating order with your hands, creates order in your mind.
- According to science, people who make their bed are happier.
- It signals your brain that details matter.
- It honors your promise to yourself.
- It promotes self-trust and confidence.

Last week, you chose one 10-minute task to do each day. You scheduled it on your calendar, and followed through no matter what. In doing that, you began to pour your foundation of self-trust. (Woot woot!!!) I also told you that the next week you'd add a second task. Making your bed every morning is the second 10-minute task. Please add it to your calendar.

The following simple tasks are the only exercise in this chapter:

- Commit to making your bed every morning.
- Put it as a task on your calendar.
- Honor your commitment.
- Allow yourself to really enjoy the process.

You can choose to grumble about the drudgery of the process, or you can choose to find joy in it. Both options are available to you.

So, you made your bed? Wahoooo! Celebrate the feeling of accomplishment. My dear friend, you deserve it! It won't be long before you're buying a fancy pillow or two just to make it look prettier, and attending to the nightstand...and organizing the dresser...and buying matching hangers for the closet...

If your budget allows, do yourself a HUGE favor and invest in really good sheets (you're welcome!), put a quilt, comforter, or duvet on your bed that makes you giggle happily, and take pleasure in running your hand over the quality fabric. Elicit joy in as many of your senses in the process as possible, and you will create an empowering habit that will trickle out and touch many, many other areas of your life in joyful, unexpected ways.

Chapter 8 – Notice Your Thoughts

"True health begins with your thoughts."
~Dr. Christiane Northrup

As I promised you in the previous chapter, now that you've got your vision, are well on your way to re-establishing self-trust, made your plan, and taken action by making your plan and working your daily 10-minute tasks, all the reasons you didn't do it in the first place will bubble up to the surface.

It may feel uncomfortable, and confusing, but, my dear, you are sitting on a goldmine for personal development that goes way, way, WAY beyond just cleaning your messy house! (Can I get a woot woot???)

Notice your thoughts and the feelings that arise from them. Write them down. Notice where you feel the thoughts in your body. Write those down too. These are gems on your path that will open the door to your transformation from messy housekeeper to clean, clutter-free, organized, creative dynamo!

Also, as I said in the previous chapter, you could spend years in therapy hoping all your subconscious beliefs will eventually drift to the surface so you can evaluate and process them as an emotional adult, or you can invite them to the surface by taking the very actions that you've avoided to keep them repressed.

Let's face it, your environment, your exterior – the people, places, and things you surround yourself with – are merely a reflection of your interior. (Yeah, I'm going to keep hammering that one home!) Paying attention to the thoughts and feelings that drive your actions and dictate your results will put you at a distinct advantage by knowing what the hell they actually are.

Children feel their feelings without filter, or even a care about the feelings of others at times. Self-control is an important skill to cultivate, but as adults, we've stuffed our feelings down for so long, and let the incessant chatter of our thoughts run rampant for so many years, that it can be difficult to get quiet enough to hear the still, small voice of your intuition.

When you pay close attention to your thoughts, you open the door to changing your fundamental beliefs, but first, you've got to get quiet enough to hear them.

Meditation

Meditation saved my life. Literally. I used to be prone to depression, but have this strange medical condition where most medications have the opposite effect on me than what they're intended for. For instance, cortisone is supposed to soothe the skin, but it breaks me out in hives that look like somebody took a blowtorch to my skin. If I want to get pregnant, all I have to do is take birth control pills and I'm as fertile as the Napa Valley. If there is a wonky, weird side effect to a medication, I'll get it.

After the birth of my daughter, I was plunged into a state of depression that lasted for two and a half years. I was afraid to get on medication for fear of the reaction, but the depression was so bad that, in desperation, I finally went to the doctor to get help.

Days 1-3 on antidepressants: I felt jittery and weird, and had strange dreams that felt very, very real.

Days 4-6 on antidepressants: Anxiety built into paralyzing panic attacks, which was something I'd never experienced before in my life and hope never to experience again.

Night 6 on antidepressants: Those strange dreams turned into hellish nightmares I could not escape from because they followed me into the next day. For the first time in my life, I actually considered committing suicide to end the torment, but there was a part of me that recognized it was the medication that caused it, and I just had to hold on long enough to ride it out.

Medication can be life-changing for some people, and I am so glad it is there for them, but it is not for me. I never took another pill to alter my mood. Not an option.

The anxiety and panic attacks stuck with me for a little while, but I knew I'd have to find another way to manage my thoughts and feelings other than medication. That's when I found meditation. Beautiful, wonderful, side-effect free meditation.

For the longest time, I found it frustrating to meditate because my mind never stopped running, and certainly never shut up. I kept on because, even amidst the frustration, I *felt* better, calmer, more in control of my body, my mind, and more connected to the world around me.

They tell you to focus on your breathing, and every time the mind drifts to bring your attention back to your breath, which, let's face it, is the worst advice in the world!

What they should tell you when you learn how to meditate is this: You're going to feel like your mind has gone crazy because it jabbers non-stop (the monkey mind); you're going to feel like it's impossible to quiet and control your mind because, when you first start meditating, it is not possible; and the reason is because *focus* is a *skill* you must nurture and develop within yourself just like any other.

Meditation is learning to focus your mind, and the only way to focus your mind is to focus it continuously, repeatedly, consistently. You build focus like you build muscle, or any other skill. There is a reason it's called a ***PRACTICE***.

Meditation allows me to step out of the drama of depression, anxiety, and panic attacks, and see myself and life with a very wide lens. Meditation allows me to observe my mind, honor and respect my emotions, focus my attention and energy, and the only side effects are calm, peace, love, compassion, and kindness.

You can't bottle that shit!

That was over twenty-seven years ago. While I don't always meditate every single day, and have even gone through phases where I didn't meditate at all for months at a time, there is a profound difference in the quality of my life when I'm in a meditation phase.

Become The Observer

The best way I know of to pay attention to your thoughts is to observe them. In order to observe them, you must cultivate the skill of getting quiet via meditation. If you do not meditate, observing your thoughts objectively will be difficult, if not impossible...

In Chapter 12, I'll go into detail about how your mind works, and why, but for now, I'm going to talk about that voice in your brain that blathers on non-stop: your ego. (ego wants to be capitalized, but I refuse to grant it the honor even if it begins a sentence!)

YOU are not those thoughts. *YOU* are the thinker who has the thoughts. The distinction is subtle, yet profound.

Have you ever watched yourself think? Have you ever listened to the shit that goes through your mind? It's perplexing to me that, no matter how many years I've meditated, the poor quality of my thoughts is STILL there. Sometimes I take my own breath away by the shallow stupidity and absolute arrogance my ego can sink to. I know that's not me, it's just an aspect of my mind that truly wants to protect me from the horrors of being eaten alive by a saber-toothed tiger.

Thank goodness my ego doesn't run the show most of the time!

Detaching from the endless chatter helps you to observe it. Once you can observe your mind, you can more objectively evaluate each thought based on its merit, take responsibility for the thoughts that impact your behavior, and let go of the thoughts that don't serve you.

Why are your thoughts so important? Because, according to the tenants of cognitive behavioral therapy, your thoughts create your feelings, your feelings dictate your actions, and...as common sense deduces...your actions drive your results.

As I stated earlier, in her book *Self Coaching 101,* Brooke Castillo even goes so far as to point out that your results will *always* prove the original thought.

Keep A Journal

In my life coaching practice, Messy Bed, Messy Head is an 8-week program, and I have my clients keep a journal of their thoughts and feelings throughout the duration of the program.

Noticing your thoughts can be an enlightening experience, no doubt, but writing them down, bringing them out into the light so you can explore their validity, is where transformation happens.

In Western society, we often get stuck in the action/results loop without bothering to address the thoughts and emotions that drove the action in the first place. It's like spitting into the wind in a hurricane. If the spit doesn't fling back into your face, it'll whirl around and smack you on the back of the head.

If you can identify the thought that causes an emotion, you can change it. If you change the emotion, you take different action. If you change your actions, you change your results.

Having said that, our society has developed a paranoid, rather pathological fear of negative emotions that drives me absolutely bonkers!

Negaphobia

My BFF, Kim, and I coined the word "negaphobia" to describe the irrational fear of all things perceived as "negative."

Scroll your Facebook feed for 30 seconds. My guess is you'll see at least 1-5 memes telling you to be positive, or to focus only on the positive, and maybe even the same number describing everything perceived as negative as being "toxic" or "bad." We've become so enamored with positivity that we almost fear anything perceived at "negative." I know people who are afraid of their negative thoughts for fear of attracting something negative into their lives.

But I have news for you that may sound blasphemous: There is no such thing as "good emotions" and "bad emotions." All emotional states are within you to serve you. Period. If you feel "bad" or "negative," it is a signal that something is wrong that you need to look at, address, and take action upon. Period. Helpful, not toxic.

Feelings that "make you feel bad" are not an indictment on *YOU*, or your character; they're simply a call to action for you to examine your thoughts, to see where the emotion is coming from. It has a message for you that is critical in your personal growth and development, but if you push it away, you'll never get the message.

What's wrong with feeling an uncomfortable feeling, anyway? Better yet, where does the discomfort come from? Not the feeling itself, but the struggle within you to suppress it, or change it, or deny it, or transmute it.

Think of a wonderful emotional event in your life: a wedding, the birth of a child, or a graduation. Go for a BIG one. Remember how amazing you felt? Remember how the joy filled you to overflowing, and you'd've done anything to stay in that peak emotional state forever, but you couldn't. Why is that?

Because strong emotion, fully felt and allowed to run its

course, dissipates of its own accord. It is only when you resist, struggle, overcome, cope, or wrestle with it that an emotion metastasizes and becomes toxic.

Think of the Yin and Yang symbol...

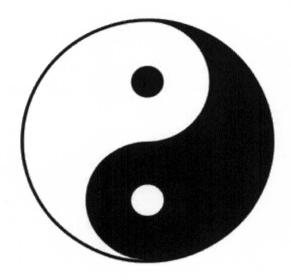

It personifies the perfection of duality by giving us contrast. Masculine and feminine. Light and dark. Night and day. Love and hate. Agony and ecstasy. Joy and despair. We are creatures of contrast, so you cannot have one without the other. Try to mute one, and you numb the other until you are emotionally colorblind.

Dissatisfaction, fear, failure, and rejection are your BEST friends. You can even use them as fuel to transform your life. (This is actually the topic of my next book, so I won't belabor the point, but suffice to say: Your feelings serve you. All feelings. All the time.)

Filters and Lenses

If you don't like the quality of your feelings, it's a call to examine your thoughts. The quality of your thoughts are dictated by your beliefs – in other words, the things you believe to be "True."

I'm a photographer, so I love the analogy that the intention you put into your thoughts serve as filters and lenses that change how you focus on your life.

Judgment and condemnation stem from offending black and white beliefs you subconsciously hold that result in harsh, punitive thoughts and create vibrations in your body which taint everything observed through that vibration with a tinge of superiority, bitterness, austerity, and resentment.

On the flip side, kindness, curiosity, and compassion create vibrations in the body that are warm, inviting, and opening. Kindness, curiosity, and compassion paint everything you examine within yourself, and the world at large, with goodness, joy, and love.

As you explore your thoughts and feelings, let kindness, curiosity, and compassion be the filters and lenses through which you view yourself and the world.

Uncover Hidden Beliefs

If it's true that thoughts create your feelings, feelings dictate your actions, and actions drive your results - which it is - then where do your thoughts come from? The quality of your thoughts is governed by your subconscious beliefs. In Chapter 12, I'll go into detail about your subconscious mind and how to change your beliefs. For now, it's important for you to understand that your subconscious beliefs 100% dictate the quality of your thoughts.

The problem: We don't know what most of our subconscious beliefs are! By definition, subconscious beliefs aren't known, or even obviously knowable. How do you find them? How can you change them?

Just as feelings leave an energetic trace, and affect everything you touch, see, feel, and do, subconscious beliefs leave a trace too. They leave clues, like tiny li'l breadcrumbs you can follow. As you go through the exercise of writing your thoughts and feeling in your journal, you'll notice common threads start to emerge.

The strong desire to feel something, or have something, is usually a signal that you don't have it already. For instance, as I went through the process of exploring my thoughts and feelings, I noticed a theme of self-worth emerge. I wanted to feel valuable, I wanted worth, I wanted to feel worthwhile. By exploring thoughts and feeling, and corresponding actions and results, I uncovered a subconscious belief of worthlessness that governed the quality of my thoughts.

Simply bringing that into the light allowed me to see it as the paper tiger it was, and, even better, it dissolved into nothingness.

Is this work? Yes! Is it easy? No. Is it worth the effort? Absolutely!

In the next chapter, I'm going to show you how to take the

subconscious beliefs you've discovered about yourself, as well as the discoveries you've made in writing your story in Chapter 4, and use them to get the leverage on yourself you need to change that messy house of yours into the home you and your family deserve to live in.

But before we dive in, let's wrap up this chapter with a quick exercise.

Journal Exercise

For the duration of this program, keep a journal to notice and document your thoughts, the feelings that arise from them, and how and where you feel them in your body.

Chapter 9 – Get Leverage On Yourself

"You will do more to avoid pain than
you will ever do to gain pleasure."
~Tony Robbins

If you want to make a permanent change to your behavior, you must get leverage on yourself. Be willing to explore why you do what you do, and why you've done what you've done, with an open heart and mind filled with kindness, curiosity, acceptance, and compassion.

It's absolutely true that love, acceptance, curiosity, and compassion form the foundation of wellness and provide the key to lasting transformation, but first, you need to blow out the cobwebs!

To get leverage on yourself, you'll need to stir up a little pain because, as Tony Robbins says, every human being is hardwired to avoid pain, and gain pleasure, while expending as little effort as necessary. This is an immutable fact of human nature you can use to your advantage.

Look, you're a fabulous person with a few bad habits, but habits can be changed. Finger-pointing, drama, and condemnation are useless endeavors that only ensure you'll feel worse about yourself as you continue the undesired behavior.

Pain, used consciously and intelligently, can drive the impetus to change, but you want to avoid getting stuck in a place of judgment and condemnation. Harsh judgment and condemnation result in victimization and blame. No good can come from either.

There is a huge difference between blame and responsibility. There is an even bigger difference between having habits that don't serve you and believing your habits are your identity.

Taking responsibility from a place of love and self-compassion means being willing to explore where you've erred so you can free yourself from the things that no longer serve you.

In this chapter, I'll show you how to use pain and pleasure intelligently to arrive at a place of peace, harmony, and love.

Personally, I discovered the joy of using pain and pleasure to change my habits back in the 90s! I bought Tony Robbins' Personal Power program for my husband for Christmas. I was super excited to give it to him, but he had no interest. (It wasn't until afterward that I realized I consciously thought I was giving him a gift, but, subconsciously, it was me I bought it for!)

I used the Personal Power program to quit smoking, but I did it by...not quitting smoking.

Confused? Let me explain...

When I decided to quit smoking, I did not put the cigarettes down. Instead, I gave myself permission to smoke as much as I wanted, with one caveat: Every time I lit a cigarette, I consciously made myself *feel* what smoking was costing me – mentally, emotionally, spiritually, financially...I hit all the pain points.

I took things that were naturally repugnant to me about smoking, and enhanced them. Oh, yeah, I made my ego an ally and put it to work creating worse case scenarios! Growing up in a messy house - smelling the clothes I picked up off of the floor to see if they were dirty or clean-ish before I got dressed for school - made me hyper aware of unpleasant scents.

That kind of stuff is primo FUEL for a bonfire! As I smoked I pictured smoke writhing around my hair, clinging to each hair shaft, so that my hair smelled like stale, putrid and nasty cigarette smoke.

Have you ever smelled the sweat of an older person who's a lifelong smoker and coffee drinker? Truly cringe worthy for me, so I pictured that hideously maleficent odor seeping from my pores! (Notice the drama in the language I'm using.)

I'm a fairly intelligent woman, and take a certain amount of pleasure and pride in that, so that was something else I chose to target. When I inhaled, I pictured gloppy, gooey tar sticking to my brain cells, leaching my intelligence away, making me stupider with every puff.

To add to my sensory misery: it was also winter time in Salt Lake City, UT, where I lived at the time. A very cold, snowy, miserable winter, and I didn't smoke inside my house because I hated the smell so much. Oh, yeah, I used my shivering bones as FUEL too!!!!

The day I quit, February 7, 1997, I sat on my back porch with a half-smoked pack of cigarettes in my hand, and said, "You will not control my life. I will not allow you to infect my life for another second." I tossed them in the trash.

If you'll notice, not once did I mistake MYSELF for being disgusting, putrid, nasty, cringe-worthy, or leaching away my intelligence. It was the cigarette and smoke that were offensive, not me. It literally took less than six weeks – no time at all in the grand scheme of things – for my brain to flip that switch, and only once have I ever looked back.

The one time was a year later, and it was because smoking is a hand to mouth habit. Over the year that followed me quitting I packed on about 70 pounds! I was so distressed about gaining weight, that I said "fuck it!" and tried to start smoking again, but couldn't do it.

I didn't just stop smoking, I changed my identity from a smoker into a non-smoker who would NEVER even consider turning to smoking a cigarette no matter how rough things were, or how fat I got. And darling, let me tell you, I've been plunged into utter despair, divorce, death, poverty, homelessness, unemployment, and it's never once occurred to me to reach for a cigarette to cope. Not once.

THAT is how you get leverage on yourself.

Each time I changed my identity I did it by...
- Exploring what the disempowering habit costs you mentally, emotionally, financially, and spiritually.
  - Write it down.
- Decide what is it specifically about the habit that grosses you out.
- Tap into your emotion. It is powerful!

- Make the cigarette, or the clutter, or the filth, or the chocolate the problem, and the source of your discomfort, not YOU.
  - My beautiful friend, don't ever confuse the problem with yourself. YOU are divine. Period. A child of God/Universe/Spirit/Source, or whatever you call that glorious creative source, and an heir to First Cause with all the rights and privileges associated with being the daughter of the creator of the universe. Just sayin'...
- Be consistent.
  - Every time you engage in the habit, twist the knife, and make the pain real. If you can muster tears, all the better!

Through engaging in this process, you can shed the illusions that produce messiness – can, in fact, never produce anything but – and embrace the woman you dream of being. The woman who would never allow her home to get out of hand lives deep inside you. You picked up this book because she's crying for your attention. Use pain and pleasure intelligently to set her free.

You can tell yourself, "I suck!" (Unintelligent, demoralizing, and no good can come of it.) Or, you can say, "This sucks!" (Intelligent, observative, and something constructive you can work with to make it not suck.)

You can tell yourself, "I'm a lazy pig!" (Unintelligent, abusive, and incredibly destructive.) Or you can tell yourself, "My house is messy, which is not a clean, safe environment for my children." (Intelligent, productive, and taking responsibility without casting blame will produce far more constructive action.)

The problem created when you use such harsh, destructive language with yourself is you'll turn around and use softeners to dull the pain when you tell yourself how much it doesn't matter – even though it really does – and bury the pain in your subconscious mind to jaundice the quality of your thoughts.

Are you sensing the vicious circle set in motion?

The Power of I Am

You've heard English author Edward Bulwer-Lytton's adage, "The pen is mightier than the sword." And almost 200 years later, his meaning is still crystal clear: Words have power.

The fact is, language is powerful, and how you use it matters. The language you use when you talk to your children will shape their little lives, for better or worse, far more than anyone else. But the language you use when you talk to yourself is most important of all because the quality of their lives comes down to the quality of yours.

When you utter the words "I am...," whatever follows is a command by the subconscious mind to bring it into reality.

If you frequently use a phrase like "I am lazy," you will never find the motivation to get up and clean your house.

If you frequently indulge in language that drains you of energy, you will be drained. If you frequently indulge in language that demoralizes you, you will be demoralized. It really is that simple.

But you can't lie to yourself either. Telling yourself "I am a fantastic housekeeper," when you need only look around the room you're in to know that statement is false, will only cause you to distrust yourself further.

You will never change if you lie to yourself, so changing your language is found in the zone of proximal development too. Use bridge language to get you to where you want to go.

Telling yourself "I want my house to be a warm, welcoming home for my family" can be a language bridge that takes you from "I am lazy" to "I am a fantastic housekeeper."

I am Lazy – turns to – I want my house to be a warm, welcoming home for my family – which will naturally evolve into you actually being a fantastic housekeeper without the need to promote yourself as such.

Writing Exercise

Something I learned 25+ years ago courtesy of Tony Robbins' Personal Power II program is this: Because you are wired to avoid pain at all costs and gain pleasure if you can, you will not change until the pain of the status quo is greater than the uncertainty of change. If you tell yourself everything is peachy, when it clearly isn't, you're not going to get any leverage on yourself to change. If you have the courage to be honest with yourself, and stir up your pain points without being cruel, you can tip the scales in your favor by making living in a messy house unbearable. So unbearable that you HAVE to clean it up to get relief.

- What do you get out of living in a messy house? (You've experienced some form of pleasure from not cleaning your house or you wouldn't live that way. What is it? Remember: Honesty without brutality.)
- What is messiness costing you and your family? (Are your children embarrassed to have friends over? How does that make you feel?)
- Why do you want to clean your house?
- What will your house look like next year, or three years, or five years from now if you don't get a handle on the messiness?
- Who will you be in the future if you don't get a handle on this? (Feel free to set your inner drama queen free to answer this one. Make it awful. Make it painful. Make living in a dirty house hurt your soul.)

Time for some personal exploration. Your assignment isn't to beat yourself up, it's to give yourself perspective, and help you get leverage on yourself to change.

There are two very powerful questions you can use to change the beliefs that govern your behavior:

1. What are you getting out of living in a messy house?
2. What is it costing you and your family?

Visualization

Hopefully, you've dug up some rather uncomfortable emotions, so let's take a moment to end this segment on a positive note.

Remember the vision you created for your home? Visualize your home now, and take yourself on a tour of it. Bring up as much detail as possible, and write it down, or paint it, or dance it.

Fill yourself up with the vision you *want* to create...

Chapter 10 – A Place For Everything

"A place for everything, everything in its place."
~Benjamin Franklin

My beautiful friend, I am so proud of you! If you've worked the program, by now you've established the habit of daily calendaring. Woot woot!!! Cause for celebration, for sure, and you're probably itching to get into the meat and potatoes of decluttering!

Your wish... is granted!

There are several ways to approach decluttering, and everybody swears their method is the only method that works permanently. Balderdash! (I've always wanted to use that word!)

There is the *category method*, which means you go through your house by categories: books, shoes, belts, kitchen gadgets, and so on.

Let's take shoes.

In the category method, you take all shoes and put them in a pile, then sort them by trash, donate, and keep. Trash goes straight into the garbage can. Donated shoes go straight into your car and taken to Goodwill, or wherever you like to donate things. The kept shoes get put away, right away.

My problem with this is it assumes your closet is already clean and putting the shoes away won't be a hassle, and that you know where all of your shoes actually are. If the closet is packed full of junk, or you've got shoes missing its mate, it most certainly will be a hassle!

There is the *room-by-room method*, which is self-explanatory. My problem with this method is stuff from that room often gets foisted off onto other rooms, and by the time you get every room done, the first room is trashed again. Everything just gets shuffled around. Way, way too exhausting!

My preferred method is the *compartment method*. It starts simple and becomes more complex: drawer by drawer, dresser by dresser, closet by closet, and then room by room. By starting small, it allows you to assign a purpose for the space – i.e., panty drawer, sock drawer, bra drawer – and assign everything that goes into that space a "home."

From that point forward, once socks have a "home" where they belong, you do not put socks in the panty drawer because...well...they don't belong there. I adore simplicity and order, so simple methods tend to work better for me than unnecessarily complex ones. If your aim is simplicity, you'll never get there by pouring complex energy on your project. Just sayin'...

Personally, I think the best way to do it is to follow your intuition. Only your intuition knows the shortest, fastest, most expedient route to creating order in *your* mind, and thus *your* home.

There is the voice in your head, the ego, and there is the *knowing* that exists beyond words that whispers to you from somewhere deep within your body. I can guarantee you it is

NOT in your brain. Check your heart, or your gut, to find your intuition. Mine is most definitely in my gut.

Are you ready? This is going to be fun!

Why Clutter Accumulates

You have a bedroom, don't you? And so do your children? You have a cupboard where you keep your dishes, right? And another where you keep your glasses? There's also a closet where you hang your clothes, isn't there?

Can we agree that a designated place to go to the toilet – one that does not change just because you don't feel like walking to the bathroom - is essential to a well-organized home?

There are two primary reasons why clutter accumulates in your house.

1. You don't have a system for processing new things that come into your dwelling.
2. Things already in your house don't have a "home."

Things that do not have a place where they belong in your home are shiftless, aimless and bring that shiftless, aimless, disorganized energy into your home.

I fought the battle with chaos and clutter for years until I learned to give all my possessions a home, and, in this chapter, I'll walk you through an exercise to create order and clarity in your home. We'll start by assigning a home to the things you love and then wrap up by getting rid of anything you don't have room for, or anything that doesn't spark peace, contentment, or joy within you.

Grab your workbook and calendar, and let's get busy!

Writing Exercise

This is an exercise in finding your intuition and getting a feel for what type of energy you want to bring into your home. Take quick impressions, the first ones that pop into your awareness, and write them down in your workbook.

Do this for each room in your house. It really shouldn't take you more than five minutes per room.

Walk into any room in your house. Close your eyes and breathe deeply.

- What do you feel emotionally? (Quick impressions.)
- Where do you feel it in your body? Is it anywhere specific, and does it have energy behind it? (The energy could be heavy, light, warm, whispery, cool, cold, or tingly, to name a few, but certainly not limited to them.)
- What do you *want* to feel when you enter the room?
- What do you think stops you from feeling it?
- How can you create the feeling you want to feel when you enter the room?

The first impression is typically your intuition. The place you felt the impression most often is typically the seat of your intuition. The part of your brain that struggles with words to define it, or needs to tell a story about it, is your ego.

A word of advice: It's going to get worse before it gets better. Much worse! You're dragging stuff out of closets, emptying drawers, creating order. I suggest you start small, and don't feel like you've got to do everything in a week. You're just setting yourself up for overwhelm and failure if you do that.

Remember to work in 10-minute tasks, and, depending on your schedule, budget your time in totally doable 10-minute tasks. If you have an hour, great, do five or six 10-minute tasks! If you have 20 minutes, fantastic, do two 10-minute tasks! You're in this for the long haul, so there's no need to rush it!

Go from room to room and take an inventory. What is trash, what gets donated, what stays, and remember, if it stays, where will it "live?" Anything that stays in your house needs to have a home.

As you go from room to room taking your inventory, make a cursory assessment of where things will live. Open each dresser drawer, and decide what lives there. Panties need a panty drawer. Socks need a sock drawer. You get the picture. Draw a rendering of your dresser and write the label on it: panty, socks. Make it official like a blueprint of your home in each room.

Are you overwhelmed and drowning in chaos and clutter because you've got too much stuff? Why do you keep all of that shit? Get rid of it! There is someone out there who'd love to have the things that don't bring you Joy.

When you sell or donate an item, take a moment to thank the item for serving your family's needs, and send a blessing that the family who finds the item will see it as a treasure and love it. I believe blessings are powerful intentions. By blessing the items before passing them on to another, you'll cultivate a grateful heart, *and* send love out into the world. It's a win-win!

Hidden Clutter

All the things in your house carry energy that creates the environment your children grow up in. The things you love carry the energy of love. The things you don't want carry that neglected, unwanted energy too.

There is the obvious stuff – laundry, dishes, and toys – that add to the energy of chaos and clutter and general messiness of your home, but there is hidden clutter too that can suck your energy until you deal with it.

Oh, you can find clutter behind the refrigerator, under the sofa, and atop the bookcase, for sure, but the #1 place for hidden clutter that sucks your energy is...drumroll...your email inbox! How many unopened emails do you have? Hundreds? Thousands? Do you have more than one email address? Better yet, when is the last time you emptied your inbox?

I did not understand the importance of how much residual energy your inbox contains until I went through mine and emptied it. Years ago, I worked for a metaphysical church. During the time I worked there, they hired a very charismatic personality to be minister, who wound up splitting the church and starting his own ministry. As a paid employee of the church who lost their job because of the deep division, I was in the loop on everything that went on. There was lots of excitement, hope, drama, and heartache that took place during that period of time, and much of it happened via email.

It wasn't until I found those emails from years earlier, and deleted them, that I realized the energetic drain they'd had on me. The moment I hit "Select All" and "Delete," I swear it felt like I lost 10 pounds of toxic sludge.

Liberating!!!

Also, how many mailing lists are you subscribed to that you don't want to be bothered with anymore? Unsubscribe!

The #2 place for hidden clutter? Your Facebook newsfeed, especially during election time! How many people are on your friends list that you don't even know, or like? What about that off-putting redneck cousin whose posts make you cringe, the super judgy political zealot who thinks everyone who doesn't believe what they do are vile pond scum, or the BFF from kindergarten you no longer have anything in common with? I highly recommend taking a hatchet to your friends list, or at least hiding those whose posts tend to drain you. Seriously.

Containers Really ARE For Hoarders

In her fantastic book *The Life-Changing Magic Of Tidying Up*, Marie Kondo makes the statement, "Containers are for hoarders."

When I first read that, I thought, "Daaaamn, that's a little judgy an' harsh!," but the more I think about it, the more I've come to believe she's absolutely right. Some things need storage: Christmas decorations, extension cords not in use, extra batteries. Things like that. But a box filled with old chargers for Nokia and Motorola cellphones you had five to 10 years ago, or that first generation iPod nano? Really?

Seems like the more storage cabinets you have, the more you need. They're never enough. Get rid of them!

Living In Joy

Einstein said it best: $E=MC^2$. What this means on a practical level that you and I can incorporate into our lives is: everything is energy, and energy is everything.

The speed of light is a scientifically measurable event. The temperature of the air, or the sun, or the moon and stars are scientifically measurable events, and so are the magnetic forces each radiate. Likewise, your brainwaves – your thoughts – are scientifically measurable events. As are your feelings and actions and results.

When you hold something in your hand, and look at it, think about it, there is a subtle vibration that wells-up from your body. If you appreciate the object, the vibration that ripples through every cell in your body is gratitude. If you don't really like the object, the vibration that ripples through every cell in your body is unhealthy stress. Not obvious stress, but draining, energetically depleting stress nonetheless.

You deserve to live in peace and harmony and joy, and your children deserve to feel safe and protected. If you are surrounded by things that you don't really like, or even want, the measurable potential of your emotions infuses the objects with that stressful, depleting energy.

Hold something you love in your hand. Notice the feelings that flow through you. They are flowing into that object too. Surround yourself with things that bring you peace, contentment, and joy. If the things in your home do none of those things, get rid of them.

Chapter 11 – What's Missing

"Character isn't something you were born with
and can't change, like your fingerprints.
It's something you weren't born with
and must take responsibility for forming."
~Jim Rohn

Without a doubt, self-honesty – the ability to look at yourself, your past and present decisions and resulting behavior, with unflinching truthfulness through the lens of curiosity, acceptance, and compassion – is the single most useful, productive, and empowering character trait you can develop within yourself. I would argue that self-honesty is the foundation upon which all true personal development progress stands upon. Without it, your house of cards would surely crumble.

I used to be the world's greatest at shining a light on the flaws of everyone around me...rather brutally too. I saw where they erred, certainly how they could've done better, but couldn't see the truth of myself at all. I thought I could, thought I did, but it was just pacifying shit my ego told me to make me feel better. (We'll go into detail on the ego in the next chapter.)

Developing the ability to engage in bonafide, compassionate self-honesty is a process that involves moving away from victimization and drama, and all the emotional charge that certain habits, behaviors, and thought processes have over you, and moving toward curious, compassionate objectivity and acceptance of yourself.

Remember, it's a process, not an epiphany!

You will not wake up one day with the ability to analyze yourself with kindness, curiosity, compassion, or objectivity, and that's okay. You don't have to pick yourself apart, but until you can ditch the victimization and drama and accept full responsibility for the condition of your home, and your life, they will never change.

Until you can look at your thoughts, feelings, actions and the results you've produced objectively – without putting an emotional charge you're not willing to experience on them – you will not make forward progress in your evolution. Period.

The path out of chaos and clutter is one in which you take responsibility for the condition of your house, and you cannot truly do that if you're not willing to be an objective observer of the life you've created to this point.

Writing Exercise

A couple of caveats before you get started:

1. Ditch the victimization and drama, and strive for fact. There's no need to bow at the confessional and spew your guts to the world. This exercise is for you, and you alone. It's meant to be clarifying and informative, not punitive.

2. Don't worry about shining the light on anybody but yourself.

Answer these questions with an open, compassionate heart

and a curious, objective mind...

- Can you look at yourself honestly without finger-pointing, wallowing in self-pity, victimization, or condemnation?
  - If not, what prevents you?
- Are you living life at your full potential?
  - What are the decisions and choices you've made that prevented you from expressing your fullest potential?
- Are you living in a home that gives you and your family a profound sense of ease, peace, and belonging?
  - What are the decisions and choices you've made that prevented you from transforming your house into a home?
- Can you pinpoint what's held you back and kept you and your family drowning in messiness all these years?

How true are your answers to these questions? Did you get an emotional charge while answering them?

Look at what you've written, and cross out any inflammatory, dramatic, judgmental language.

Here's an example. I can say, "I'm tall." This may not seem like judgmental language, but it actually is because, while height is factual, tallness or shortness is subjective. Tall in relation to whom, or what? To a class of first graders? Yes, I'm tall. To an NBA team? Not so much. Factually, I'm 5'9". There's no need to add or subtract language from it.

I could also answer the second question with something completely disempowering like, "I wouldn't know my full potential if it bit me on the ass!" Or, "Not even close!"

While those might be completely true, it's not super helpful, is it? Not when a simple "No, because I haven't taken the time to examine what that means to me yet" is factual, but not punitive.

Character Building

We think that by the time we're adults we're supposed to have this whole life/adulting thing all figured out, but increasingly, that isn't the case.

(Please, please, PLEASE, do not do this part until you've mastered the art of compassionate, objective self-honesty. You'll only wind up beating yourself into the ground, and that is not productive at all!)

Here's the good news: With exercise, you can build muscle at any age; with reading, you can build intellect at any age; with meditation, you can quiet your mind at any age; and, with practice, you can build character at any age.

Wahooooo!!!

Integrity is important. Character matters. Now that you've got an understanding of how important it is to employ self-honesty to look at yourself with curiosity and compassion, it's time to look at your character flaws. There's at least one that is blocking your path, and it's likely a logjam behind which all your creativity and potential lay still and silent and unexpressed.

What is a logjam? Back in the day, timber was thrown in a river and floated downstream to the mill. Occasionally, there'd be a blockage on the river, a logjam, that caused everything behind it to pile up. Your forward progress can be stopped by a single, or just a few, areas of weakness, but when you cultivate self-honesty, it helps you identify what's missing so you can accept it and take responsibility for it, because only then will you be able to rectify it.

I used to pride myself on my spontaneity. There was no need to "get ready" because I had a go button. Push it, and I was out the door and on my way in under five minutes. I thought I was "going with the flow," but after decades of not really gaining traction in my career because I drifted wherever the wind blew me, I came to understand that there is something to be said for structure, and there is a big difference between being in Universal Flow and drifting aimlessly.

When I looked at myself closely, one major character flaw that held me back and kept me from progressing forward in my life, stood head and shoulders above the rest: self-discipline. The simple fact is, I'd never bothered to cultivate self-discipline within myself.

For several frustrating years, I tried and tried to institute structure in my life, but it kept falling apart and never really worked for me. Turns out, I had to master the art of self-honesty before I went through the process of personal evaluation to find the missing link within myself.

Once I mastered self-honesty, self-discipline became the logjam that kept me small and silent and blocked my ability to get into the flow of life. And even then, it took a series of trials and errors before I realized the thing I lacked, which I couldn't move forward without, was self-discipline.

If your home is not the place you want it to be, and if you

are not who you want to be, it is because there is a logjam within you. Some essential character trait that you are missing. There is no shame in it! Once you find it, and rectify it by developing that trait within yourself, you will break free of all the things that hold you back and keep you stuck in clutter and chaos and messiness, and it'll liberate your creativity in ways you cannot even imagine right now!

Can I get a WAHOOOOO?!?

List o' Character Traits

We all have a list of character flaws, which is only helpful in determining what positive character traits you want to develop within yourself. It's merely informative and should never be used as a weapon to beat yourself down with. Otherwise, throw it in the trash!

Here is a list of a few positive character traits you might wish to develop within yourself. These are all marvelous, overlapping qualities that build upon each other and are something you can certainly strive for, and, surprisingly, it takes less time than you may realize to develop them within yourself.

- Conscientiousness**
- Self-honesty
- Self-discipline
- Integrity
- Loyalty
- Grit/Perseverance
- Responsibility
- Compassion
- Humility
- Generosity
- Fairness
- Respect
- Kindness
- Thoughtfulness
- Reliability
- Politeness

- Openness
- Agreeableness
- Assertiveness
- Optimism

**According to an article in Frontiers of Psychology by Angela L. Duckworth, et al, of all the character traits listed, conscientiousness is the single biggest predictor of success.

Self-Discipline Challenge

I'm going to call this the Self-Discipline Challenge, but feel free to insert any character trait you wish to develop within yourself! As I stated earlier, I had to develop self-honesty within myself before I could develop self-discipline.

First, I'll show you what my Self-Discipline Challenge looked like, then we'll talk about how you can create your challenge to meet your specific needs...

Heading into middle age, I have a spinal cord injury (bruised, not severed) and recently received a diagnosis of borderline diabetes. Knowing that, I am going to have to lose weight to get healthy (such an endeavor has been the bane of my existence as an adult, but it's no longer a wish or a hope, it's a necessity) so I can halt and reverse the relentless march of a progressive disease before it's too late. There is no way that can happen if I don't develop self-discipline.

This is what I decided to do to change my path and move toward health, rather than eventual decline and decay...

1. I did NOT go on a diet!!! (Unlike the THOUSANDS of other diets I'd started on and failed. If you want a different result, do things differently than you've habitually done them.)

2. I recognized I needed to create a track record of success, which was the one thing I did not have, and failing at yet another diet sure as shit wouldn't give me. I had lots of references to support my inner feeling that I "never see things through" – countless diets I'd failed at, and tons of projects I'd started and never finished – but precious little success to call upon.

3. I found a 30-day challenge that had absolutely NOTHING to do with weight loss or health or fitness or exercise, or any other buzzword associated with the diet and exercise industry. It was a 30-day gratitude/visualization challenge, and I decided that, no matter what, I was going to do it each and every day...even on the days it sucked. (And yes, even gratitude can suck when your ego starts to make excuses on days 14-24, which mine certainly did!)

4. When the suck kicked in on days 14-24, because my old habits felt threatened, I focused on how much worse I'd feel if I gave into the pressure and gave up. I'd have to live with my disappointment and make the same tired old excuses for myself that I'd done for years, and that was absolutely untenable! When I felt myself weaken, I consciously harnessed the power of my inner drama queen to make the thought of giving up even more painful. (A consciously twisted knife in your own heart aimed at your own weakness is a super useful tool!)

5. On day 30, I felt confident and accomplished and celebrated my success!!!

6. On day 31, I looked for my next challenge because I discovered that:
    a. I can do ANYTHING for 30 days!
    b. But, most importantly, I actually CAN discipline myself to meet a challenge, which is something I now LOVE to do!)

Don't get caught up in the challenge because it's not about gratitude (although a thankful heart certainly helps). It's about *self-discipline*...or whatever character trait you're working on at the moment.

To develop any character trait, be willing to explore:

- What it is
- What it means to you
- How you behaved in the past that robbed you of this trait
- How you will behave in the future to develop this trait

Your Challenge
- Create a track record of success. A simple 30-day challenge targeted directly at the character trait you wish to develop is a wonderful place to start.
- Keep it simple! A 5-minute-a-day gratitude challenge, something that develops appreciation without overwhelming you, is a good starting place. (While they certainly have their place in personal development; in the beginning, no couch to 5K programs, please!)
- Make it something you will actually do.
- Put it on your calendar!

- Do not break trust with yourself!

Before you begin, here's a meditation for you.

Get the character trait you want to develop clear in your mind...

What will your life look like in 1, 3, 5, 10 years if you don't develop this character trait? Picture it vividly, generate strong feelings of disappointment within yourself at the possibility of failure, then consciously use it as fuel every time your will starts to weaken.

Next, imagine what your life will look like in 1, 3, 5, 10 years if you develop this character trait now. Picture it vividly, generate strong feelings of accomplishment, authentic pride, and optimism within yourself, then consciously use it as fuel every single day as you complete your challenge.

Chapter 12 – Explore Your Mindset

"Failing to understand the workings of one's
own mind is bound to lead to unhappiness."
~Marcus Aurelius

You've done it! If your house isn't sparkling clean, you're well on your way to orderliness nirvana! You deserve a hearty WAAAAHHHHOOOOO!!!! (Doing the Snoopy dance for you!)

Your drawer, closet – maybe even your whole house – is looking good. You're feeling good, sparkly rainbows shoot from your rooftop, and unicorns graze on your lawn.

No? Mine either.

The #1 secret of the Universe: Now that you've got your vision, plan, and action set in motion, you'll face inevitable stumbling blocks. Consider the possibility that these stumbling blocks are gifts from the Universe. Really, I swear they are!

I don't want to bust that warm, fuzzy glow of accomplishment, but reality beckons. When it comes to cleaning, decluttering, and organizing your home, you're going to bump into two obstacles if you want to keep it that way:

1. You've trained your children, partner, and family to be slobs, and they are not going to like change.
2. Your own mind.

If your children are young, you are in the best of all positions. Young children will fuss at a new schedule for a week or so, but, with firm consistency on your part, they will soon love the order and blossom in the environment you create in your home.

Older children love to be your special helper and can be your greatest asset, or your biggest stumbling block. The trick with older children is to make cleaning your home an adventure you'll all share together, and put them to work.

Don't be afraid to delegate chores to your children. They learn everything they will ever know about keeping a clean, safe, healthy environment from you. They develop their work ethic at a surprisingly early age and need responsibility to flourish.

Teenagers? Yikes! Mine were teenagers when I finally hit my groove and started creating order. My oldest son and daughter are naturally tidy, were completely embarrassed by the messy state of our home, and were all aboard the order train. They thrived in an atmosphere of order and finally had an opportunity to blossom. It was beautiful.

My second son and my husband? Not so much. Truthfully, it was a battle. There were additional challenges with my second son that extended far beyond the chaotic state of our house, which exacerbated the hostility. I wound up "compromising" to keep peace by confining the mess to his bedroom and keeping the door closed. As long as I couldn't see it, or smell it, I could pretend it didn't exist.

Here's an unfortunate fact of life: problems not confronted and dealt with directly have an annoying way of coming back to bite you in the ass.

As of the writing of this book, my younger son is seriously injured and unable to work, so he and his family live with us. I deeply, DEEPLY regret taking the coward's way out with him as a teenager because he is still a slob. At 54, after 12 years of glorious order, I currently find myself engaged in a battle with chaos, clutter, and disorder that I didn't clean up years ago. My bad.

To get through the chaos and clutter and obstacles, you must draw healthy boundaries, which is definitely easier said than done. I used to think that drawing boundaries meant that I dictate how others will behave, but that's not the case at all! Drawing healthy boundaries does not tell people how to behave but informs them how *you'll* behave if they cross the line.

When it comes to establishing healthy boundaries, I am very much a work in progress.

Stick to your guns, insist on respect, and family can be retrained. But the biggest stumbling block you'll encounter is yourself, and your own thought process. Your mind can truly be your biggest ally, or your worst enemy.

Habits

Have you ever wondered why we have habits? Good habits, bad habits, clean habits, dirty habits. We are all, without exception, habituated beings governed by our habits. I know we'd all like to think that we're rebels, and the only exception to the rule, but we're not.

Human beings are an anomaly in the natural kingdom in that we have few evolutionary advantages, yet we, as apex predators, sit at the top of the food chain. The flourishing of our species is puzzling because we have no fur to keep us warm and dry in inclement weather, no claws for self-defense, or fangs for eating. But we have two advantages: We sweat, which enables us to regulate our body temperature; and we have the prefrontal cortex, which allows us to think, discern, analyze, observe, and grow. It is the seat of our cognitive development, personality expression, planning, willpower, decision-making – to name just a few of its functions – but, as my proofreader Sarah so aptly pointed out, it tortures us with ego's nonstop chatter too.

Neuroscience has discovered you only have so much willpower and/or creative energy per day, so it behooves our species to save as much willpower and creative energy as possible because you never know when T-Rex, or saber-toothed tiger may be stalking you!

As such, your brain analyzes patterns of behavior repeated over and over again, and relegates these actions to a different part of the brain called the basal ganglia, so it can conserve your precious willpower/creative energy in case of emergency.

In his masterful book, *The Power of Habit*, Charles Duhigg says, "You can do these complex behaviors without being mentally aware of it at all, and that's because of the capacity of our basal ganglia: to take a behavior and turn it into an automatic routine." Routine doesn't require willpower, or creative energy.

Good habits are super duper helpful, and made life for our ancestors run smoothly. They work amazingly well for us too! If you had to think of every step you must take to get through the day, you'd use up all your creative energy and be mentally exhausted by the time you finished brushing your teeth in the morning.

But bad habits? The brain's primary goal is to keep you alive in any given moment. To do that, it is wired to avoid pain and gain pleasure while expending as little energy as possible in case of emergency. You are wired to survive, not thrive. Period.

The good thing about that is, the part of your brain that governs habits is unbiased in that it will take ANY repetitive action/behavior and turn it into a habit.

The bad thing about that is, the part of your brain that governs habits is unbiased in that it will take ANY repetitive action/behavior and turn it into a habit. Just sayin'...

Anatomy of a Habit

Here is how a habit breaks down: cue, action, reward.

Think of a cue as a subconscious trigger that incites a particular chain reaction in your brain that elicits a particular action in anticipation of a specific reward. A smoker, for instance, might crave a cigarette after a meal because they've grown accustomed to having one, and feel a sense of pleasure when they do, or they may experience a sense of anxiety if the behavior loop is not completed. The last bite of the meal, then, becomes the cue.

Since most are familiar with the Pavlovian response, let's use that as an example. Ivan Pavlov did an experiment with dogs wherein he let the dogs get really hungry, then fed them while ringing a bell. He did this over and over again until, when the dogs heard the bell, they salivated because they anticipated food. They'd been conditioned to associate the bell with food, even though the two had nothing to do with each other.

When we are living on autopilot, humans are habituated, conditioned creatures who are, in actuality, no different than Pavlov's dogs. That includes me. And yes, my beautiful friend, it includes you too.

Here's the rub: Often, we become so automated that we don't even know what our cues are. I invite you to explore your habits, discover your triggers, and notice the reward you get from the action you take. The best way to change a habit is to keep the cue and the reward, and then change the action.

Habits are super-efficient energy saving behavior loops, but they are so super duper effective that they lead you toward mindlessness. And mindlessness, when you're trying to understand your thoughts, feelings, and subconscious beliefs to take control of your mind is a problem. A big problem!

Your Mind

While I am not a neuroscientist, or psychologist, I study the mind. I read everything I can get my hands on about neuroscience, evolutionary biology, psychology, spiritually, and metaphysics because, for so many years, I felt broken and completely fucked up. I needed to understand the mechanics of psychology and physiology, so I could fix myself. In addition to my English and Creative Writing studies, I took virtually every course I could get my hands on in college to understand how the mind and body function on the cellular level. (I do not know of another English major with 44 hours of pre-med centric science credits beside myself.) My understanding of the mind is on both a scientific and metaphysical plane, and I have come to understand myself on a deep level by exploring how my mind works. I'd like to share my understanding with you.

Please feel free to take what works for you and discard what doesn't, but open your mind to the possibility that you are an infinitely powerful being with the potential to create anything you wish by properly harnessing that magnificent power that lay between your ears.

There are many, many theories on the human mind, but I prefer a Jungian understanding of the psyche, with all of its archetypes, and selves, and shadows. That's way, way too complex for the purposes of this book, so I'll simplify and put it in common vernacular.

ego (Yeah, I know it's a heading, but I still refuse to capitalize it!)

That voice in your head that blathers non-stop is your ego. It warns you of impending doom, creates scenarios that feel so real, but rarely come to fruition. Its purpose is to protect you, and it is vital to your survival. If you are in danger, a well-developed ego will save your life. The problem is disaster is really rare. Like, once, or twice in a lifetime rare. The rest is just drama ego creates to feel useful because the saber-toothed tiger is no longer hanging out in the oak tree ready to pounce on you, and T-Rex isn't waiting around the corner for a snack to unwittingly stroll past.

An unoccupied ego, which is its destructive aspect, has a need for control and self-importance. Observe your mind when your unoccupied ego prattles on, and you will be horrified at some of the thoughts that drift through your head. ego is primitive, instinctual, and a ruthlessly judgmental little fucker. Don't confuse the thoughts in your head for YOU. It's not you, just an unoccupied ego literally making shit up.

ego's need for self-importance and control can easily turn pathological. When not saving your life from imminent disaster, the ego is a liar, a trickster, an overwrought drama queen, and, in my humble opinion, the devil herself is a metaphor for the ego. (In all the holy cannons, there is nothing that is said of the devil that is not also true of the human ego. Nothing.)

When you embark upon the path to change, ego will offer all sorts of opinions about why you can't do something, point out all of your vast number of flaws, but when you keep going, the ego will change its tune by offering you reasons that seem totally reasonable and valid, but send you on a merry chase trying to find your tail. Or a vast litany of reasons, which don't actually exist.

You know those thoughts I'm talking about...

Remember that time your auntie smacked your hand when you reached for the cookie, so now you hide cookies under your bed?

Could it be the trauma that keeps you from progressing in your career?

That's your ego sending you down blind alleys, and leading you a merry chase, just so it can lead the way to be your savior.

Conscious Mind

The part of your mind that is under your direct control is the conscious mind. You can observe your ego, with all its histrionics, via the conscious mind, and consciously choose to direct ego toward more productive endeavors. The conscious mind weighs, measures, analyzes, and discerns, and is the seat of our intellect. Properly harnessed, the conscious mind has dominion over the ego; and is the vehicle you will use to create your vision, set a goal, draw up a plan, take action, observe your thoughts, evaluate your beliefs, get leverage on yourself, and produce results.

Subconscious Mind

The subconscious mind is the seat of control for all of the billions, if not trillions, of functions going on in every cell of your body in any given moment, and it is not under your control. (It is also the bridge between the physical and spiritual worlds, but that's a topic for another book.)

Because the subconscious mind is unbiased and completely amenable to suggestion, any suggestion, people think the subconscious mind is dumb and programmable, but the fact is, without the intervention of the conscious mind, your subconscious mind received the vast majority of its programming before the age of 7.

Jung says that once the subconscious mind accepts something as TRUE – whether it is factual or not is irrelevant – it will go to war with any suggestion that opposes it. Why do you think people have such a nearly pathological need to be right that they would kill a fellow human being in the name of their God, or politics, or any other belief they hold to be "True?"

Beliefs

Everything you believe to be true is only true because, at one time – most likely a long before your conscious memories were even formed – somebody said something with a voice of authority, and your subconscious mind accepted it as "TRUTH." Everything. That holds true for your thoughts about yourself, as it does for your political philosophy, and your religious dogma, too.

This means that the beliefs you hold sacred might not even be your own, but muckety-muck you inherited from your family, extended family, community of birth, or even a random TV show that may have been playing in the background while your mother rocked you to sleep.

Perhaps it's possible, but I don't believe in "programming" your subconscious mind as an adult. (Such an egoic notion because ego likes to think it can because it loves the power and control, but I am not convinced.) However, I do believe you can, and should, explore and examine your beliefs, and challenge them often if necessary, to see if they still make sense.

Simply looking at something within yourself and asking the question "Is this true?" and consciously looking for all the situations in which it isn't, can be enough to dissolve subconscious barriers that do not serve you, or your family. Looking at stubborn beliefs and asking "Is there another circumstance in which this is not true?" can bring down a lot of disempowering beliefs.

Human beings are wired to survive, not thrive. (Repetitive? Yes. Truth? Absolutely!) We've come into an era of human development where we must evolve into the next, best version of ourselves, and we can only do that by going off autopilot, and taking control of our minds and mindsets.

Rituals

Rituals are tasks you perform in a specific order that elevates the mindlessness of mundane habits into mindful ceremonies. You can have habits, or you can take it to a whole other level and have rituals.

My grandmothers had rituals that governed their days, and taught me the importance of mindfulness and intention decades before it became a thing.

For instance, I take a steamy hot bath each evening. It takes several minutes to fill it up, so I get the water started, add the bath salts, or essential oil to my water, then go with my husband while I'm waiting for the tub to fill. We chat about whatever comes to mind, nothing weighty, or I work a puzzle on my iPad, and usually, I get so engrossed in whatever I'm doing that he has to remind me my bathwater is still running. I enjoy a good soak, then lather up. I always start with my face and work my way down to my feet. I love the warmth of the water, and the silky/scratchy feel of the lathered-up loofa as it glides across my skin. I take the time to breathe deeply, bless and appreciate every inch on my body, and make it a truly mindful experience. Bath-time is a ceremony for me that triggers my brain to power down, and prepare for sleep.

In the winter, when I get out of the tub, I turn on the electric blanket, so the bed will be toasty warm when we crawl beneath the covers in an hour, or so.

Creating rituals to govern your homemaking is critically important to taking a messy house, and creating the ease, peace, and safety that transform a house into a home.

Rituals elevate the monotonous to the holy.

Because rituals are so intimate and deeply personal, I encourage you to look at the rituals you engage in, and decide...

- Do they serve you?
- Do they elevate you?
- Or are you on auto-pilot?

Where Does Clutter Come From?

My wish in publishing this book is that you come to understand that – by simply tweaking your habits by choosing beliefs and thoughts and actions that serve your desire to create a home your children are proud to invite friends over to, and elevating your habits to the status of conscious rituals – you can pivot away from clutter and chaos, and set yourself, and your family free.

Hopefully, by now you understand that clutter comes, of course, from you. Your disempowering habits, and unmanaged mind can produce little else.

It may seem disheartening at first, but the moment you begin to look at the situation honestly, and take responsibility for it, you begin to understand that you are the ultimate creator of your life, and you can, in fact, create anything you want.

How Do You Clean It Up?

If your disempowering habits and chaotic mind produce messiness; conscious rituals, and taking responsibility for managing your thoughts and beliefs will produce order. It really is that simple. As I said earlier, you can go to therapy for years hoping your subconscious beliefs will eventually surface, or you can invite them to the surface by taking the actions you've avoided to keep them suppressed in the first place.

Chapter 13 – Evolution

"It is not the strongest of the species that
survive, nor the most intelligent, but
the one most responsive to change."
~Charles Darwin

You finished!!!! WOOT WOOT!!!!! WAHOOOOOOO!!!!! Go girlfriend, go girlfriend, go, go, GO GIRLFRIEND!!!

I hope you're as proud of yourself as I am proud of YOU!!! You have just been through a process that has the power to, not only clean your house, but to clear away the chaos and clutter in your mind, which will ensure that it you can keep your home clean, organized, and tidy from this point forward.

If that doesn't deserve a celebration, I don't know what does! (I want to put a whole string of dancing and celebratory emojis here, but don't think they'll survive the conversion from Word to Kindle.)

Let's go over what you learned...

- Write your history, so you can understand the forces that drove and shaped you, and get an insight into why you do what you've done. Until you understand who you are, and why you're that way, you cannot take responsibility of them. Once you take responsibility for something you can change it.
- Creating a vision what you want is, in essence, drawing a map to it. A map that gives your brain a

direction to go it. But first, you need to get a sense of what you like, and why you like it.

- There is no promise that is more important than the promise you keep to yourself. You can set goals until the cows come home, but if you don't schedule it, and honor the schedule, it is unlikely to get done. We brainstormed 10-minute tasks to bring your vision to life, put one on the calendar, and honored your calendar faithfully. You learned how important self-honesty, kindness, and compassion are.

- You built upon the daily 10-minute task by making your bed every morning, so you can start your day with a BIG win!

- You learned how your beliefs generate the quality of your thoughts; your thoughts create your feelings; your feelings dictate your actions; your actions drive your results; and that you can change your results by monitoring your thoughts, so you can choose better ones.

- People will not change until the pain of the status quo is greater than the uncertainty of change. Knowing that basic human wiring will allow you to use it to your advantage. Knowing your pain-points will allow you to get enough leverage on yourself to tip the pain scale in favor of change.

- You learned the importance of giving your possessions a home, and having a plan in place to process new items coming into your home.

- Character matters, and if you find a character trait you haven't developed within yourself, it's never too late to develop it. Never!
- You learned how your mind works, so you can use it to your advantage to change anything you want to change about yourself.

Empowering stuff!!!

You, my beautiful friend, are a magical, magnificent Being capable of creating anything you want. Yes, anything, and that includes crafting a beautiful home that is a welcoming oasis of safety and security for your family.

Once you come down off of the accomplishment high, you may size up other stumbling blocks in your life, and scoff at the page, but it's true. Now, you have a process to move through chaos and clutter to embody the organized, ingenious dynamo you were created to be, but also any other stumbling block you may face! (And yes, my beautiful friend, there will always be stumbling blocks on the way to any goal!)

The structure of the coaching process I created for Messy Bed, Messy Head – the one you just underwent – is the one I've used in my own life to evolve beyond the megaliths that stood in my path: smoking, heights, public speaking, hellish childhood, money blocks, trauma, and, of course, keeping a messy house. It is the coaching process I use for my coaching clients to help them transform their lives, and reveal their true identities too.

In fact, every book I write, every coaching program I create, will incorporate these elements in the structure of the program:

- History
- Vision
- Self-honesty, Self-trust, Self-examination
- Responsibility
- Goal setting
- Calendaring
- Planning
- Taking action w/in the Zone of Proximal Development
- Building character
- Understanding Mind

All of this is designed to cut through the mental chaos and clutter, strip away the beliefs and thoughts that keep you small, and reveal the precious gem that is authentically YOU.

If you worked this program thoroughly, you are all set to clean your house, and not be afraid to invite family and friends over to celebrate your success! But if you want to take this to a deeper level, I'm here for you. Messy Bed, Messy Head is a live coaching program I facilitate 3 times a year that starts on March 1st, August 1st, and November 1st. If you'd like to sign-up to take this deep-dive with me, and a few other like-minded ladies, I'd be honored to coach you through this material. Simply go to my website https://www.cindylcooley.com/coaching/messybedmessyhead and apply.

I am so grateful you chose me to be your mentor/guide on your journey through chaos and clutter into clean, organized, and tidy, and would love for you to share your experience with me on social media. In addition to my website https://www.cindylcooley.com/ you can also find me on Facebook at https://www.facebook.com/cindylousmuse/. Feel free to stop by and share pics of your home transformation with me, and the rest of our beautiful Facebook peeps!

Not sure about life coaching, and want to check it out? Come over to https://www.cindylcooley.com/work-with-me/ and sign-up for a FREE mini-coaching session. I'd love, love, LOVE to partner with you to find creative solutions to the stumbling blocks left in your path.

Thank you for giving me the high honor of reading my book, and working through this process to create a home that you, your husband, and your children will be excited to share with your family and friends.

I can't wait to see your fabulous home transformations on social media!

About The Author

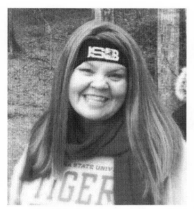 Life Coach & Transformation Strategist Cindy L. Cooley grew up in a messy house, and carried that unhealthy family tradition into adulthood for a number of years until she discovered the freedom, clarity, and balance that comes with living in a state of simplicity and order.

Cindy is a pragmatist, who is known for her straight-talk. Indeed, she looks at herself, and the world, with openness, unapologetic vulnerability, and unflinching candor. She began work to overcome her fear of public speaking at the age of 52, and recently earned Toastmasters' highest award: Distinguished Toastmaster. She is a personal development blogger, hosts the *Beautifully Joyfully You* podcast and YouTube channel, and holds a BA in Creative Writing from the University of Colorado – Boulder.

On her website https://www.cindylcooley.com/ you'll find a wealth of content, and coaching programs all created to empower you to embrace your beauty, discover your bliss, and, most importantly, to love and accept yourself as the magnificent human being you already are.

Cindy lives with her beloved husband on acreage in the middle of cow pastures and sugarcane fields just outside of Baton Rouge, Louisiana.

Made in the USA
Monee, IL
18 November 2019